Instructor's Manual

to Accompany

Medical-Surgical Nursing:
An Integrated Approach

Instructor's Manual

to Accompany

Medical-Surgical Nursing:
An Integrated Approach

Lois White, RN, PhD
Gena Duncan, RN, MSEd, MS

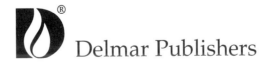

Delmar Publishers

an International Thomson Publishing company I(T)P

Albany • Bonn • Boston • Cincinnati • Detroit • London • Madrid
Melbourne • Mexico City • New York • Pacific Grove • Paris • San Francisco
Singapore • Tokyo • Toronto • Washington

COPYRIGHT © 1998
By Delmar Publishers
a division of International Thomson Publishing Inc.

The ITP logo is a trademark under license.

Printed in the United States of America

For more information, contact:

Delmar Publishers
3 Columbia Circle, Box 15015
Albany, New York 12212-5015

International Thomson Publishing Europe
Berkshire House
168-173 High Holborn
London, WC1V 7AA
England

Thomas Nelson Australia
102 Dodds Street
South Melbourne 3205
Victoria, Australia

Nelson Canada
1120 Birchmount Road
Scarborough, Ontario
Canada, M1K 5G4

International Thomson Editores
Campos Eliseos 385, Piso 7
Col Polanco
11560 Mexico D F Mexico

International Thomson Publishing GmbH
Konigswinterer Strasse 418
53227 Bonn
Germany

International Thomson Publishing Asia
221 Henderson Road
#05-10 Henderson Building
Singapore 0315

International Thomson Publishing—Japan
Hirakawacho Kyowa Building, 3F
2-2-1 Hirakawacho
Chiyoda-ku, Tokyo 102
Japan

1 2 3 4 5 6 7 8 9 10 XXX 03 02 01 00 99 98 97

Library of Congress Card No. 97-17371
ISBN: 0-8273-7680-4

Contents

Introduction

This instructor's manual is a companion to *Medical-Surgical Nursing: An Integrated Approach*. It begins with a chapter that offers suggestions on how to work with the content in Chapter 37, Critical Thinking on Multiple Systems. This chapter has been placed first since the critical thinking exercises from Chapter 37 may be used at any point in your course. This manual also includes suggested answers to the case studies and answers to all of the review questions from the text. Included in this instructor's manual is a list of resources related to the content of each chapter. These may be distributed to the students, who can use them to perform research or for extra information. Finally, a selection of transparency masters appears at the end of this manual for classroom use.

In addition to this manual, a study guide and computerized test bank are also available with *Medical-Surgical Nursing: An Integrated Approach*.

CHAPTER 37

Guidelines for Instructors in Using Critical Thinking Exercises

Critical thinking involves finding facts, sorting pertinent information, analyzing information, and applying solutions to problems. The purpose of critical thinking exercises is to develop critical thinking skills in students.

The case study critical thinking exercises in Chapter 37 can be completed alone, in a study group, or in a classroom setting. Once the case studies have been completed, have the students share their answers and charts with the entire group to enhance the learning experience. The critical thinking exercises can be used as take-home assignments for students to do on an individual basis or as group assignments. They are excellent for take-home exams to evaluate the effectiveness of student's assimilation of concepts presented in theory. Students can also present case study critical thinking exercises in the classroom setting so the entire group can experience a critical thinking opportunity. This provides variety in the classroom presentation after covering a difficult section. Critical thinking exercises work well when individual students or groups of students present the case study in post-conference.

It is important for you to have an open mind when assisting students to think critically. It does not matter how students design their diagrams, maps, or charts, as each student or group of students may arrive at or present the answers in a different manner. The important thing is that students show relationships between ideas and concepts presented in their diagrams. The process one takes in finding the answer is less important than the opportunity to use critical thinking skills, as long as sound, logical nursing judgment is used in obtaining an appropriate answer. When students are able to analyze relationships and explain concepts, critical thinking skills have been learned. Critical thinking and problem-solving skills will then become more natural in clinical experiences where decisions are made every minute.

The diabetes mellitus and cirrhosis critical thinking exercises could be used after these subjects have been covered in the curriculum. The hypertension, congestive heart failure, and chronic renal failure critical thinking exercises could be covered after each of these topics has been covered in the curriculum.

Students are encouraged to think freely and creatively. By giving specific diagram examples, some of the creativity and learning is stifled. However, students may be hesitant at first to do the maps and instructor guidance may be needed in developing and using patho-flow diagrams, concept mapping, and interrelatedness charts. Therefore, examples have been provided to assist in developing critical thinking with the use of diagrams, maps, and charts. An example of a concept map developed by a student, Cortney DeWitt, has been provided as an example (see Figure 1).

In assisting the student in developing the patho-flow map, you could first start by having the student complete a grid of the pathophysiology, diagnostic studies, signs and symptoms, and nursing interventions for the disease (see Table 1, page 4, Table 2, page 14, and Table 3, page 16). Then have students develop a patho-flow map, concept map, or interrelationship chart as appropriate.

CRITICAL THINKING EXERCISE WITH DIABETES MELLITUS

Mr. Phillips, a forty-six-year-old insurance salesman, is admitted to the hospital with the diagnosis of insulin dependent diabetes mellitus (IDDM).

- List the etiological risk factors for IDDM.
  - **family history of diabetes**
  - **exposure to environmental factors**
  - **history of gestational diabetes**
  - **history of impaired glucose tolerance**

- Brainstorm subjective and objective data that would be included in the assessment of Mr. Phillips.
  - **Subjective:** **fatigue**
    weakness
    polydipsia
    polyphagia
    familial history
    overall health status

CONCEPT MAP

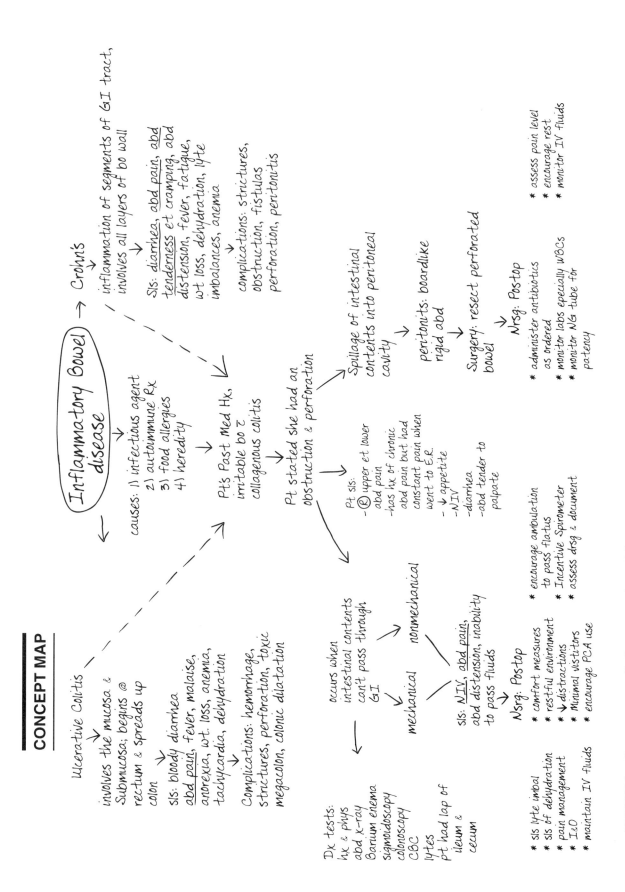

FIGURE 1   Concept map of inflammatory bowel disease. Courtesy of Cortney DeWitt.

> numbness or tingling of arms or legs
> vision problems (especially blurred vision)
> increased appetite
> **Objective:** weight changes
> mental status changes
> polyuria
> dependent redness or cyanosis of extremities
> loss of hair on lower extremities
> capillary refill

- Develop a patho-flow diagram identifying the symptoms Mr. Phillips may have been experiencing on admission and relate the pathophysiology of diabetes mellitus to the symptoms (see the examples of a patho-flow diagram in Figure 37-1 on page 1080 of the core textbook and an interrelationship chart in Figure 37-2 on page 1081 of the core textbook).

  Symptoms Mr. Phillips may have been experiencing on admission are:

thin/weight loss	**polyuria**	**polydipsia**
polyphagia	**ketoacidosis**	

  In assisting the student in developing the patho-flow map, the instructor could first start by having the student complete a grid of the pathophysiology, diagnostic studies, signs and symptoms, and nursing interventions for diabetes mellitus (see Table 1). Then have students develop a patho-flow map of the action of insulin in the body. These will all vary. An example of this is given in Figure 2. Also refer to Figure 30-2 on page 828 in the core textbook. Then have students develop a patho-flow diagram of what happens in the body when insulin is not produced in adequate amounts or is not utilized (see Figure 2). Again, Figure 2 is only an example and does not need to be reproduced exactly by the students. Encourage variety and creativity and analyze the relationships indicated by the student's map to see if they are correct.

  A patho-flow diagram developed by a student, Davette Kessel, could also be used with this exercise (see Figure 4). Figure 4 is a completed example. The instructor may wish to use a partially blank form for students to complete as provided in Figure 5.

- What diagnostic tests could the physician have ordered to confirm the diagnosis of diabetes mellitus?

  fasting blood sugar
  two hour postprandial glucose
  glucose tolerance test
  glycosylated hemoglobin

- Relate the possible results of the diagnostic tests to the pathophysiological cause of the results on the patho-flow diagram.

  All blood glucose levels would be elevated on FBS, 2hPPBS, GTT and glycosylated hemoglobin tests because of decreased insulin production or an inability to utilize insulin in the body. Also refer to Figure 3.

- If Mr. Phillips had been diagnosed with NIDDM, how would the pathophysiology and nursing care vary?

  The major contributing factor for NIDDM is obesity. In NIDDM, the pancreas is not able to meet the insulin needs of the body and/or possibly the number of insulin receptor sites are decreased or ineffective. There is enough insulin to prevent fat breakdown and ketoacidosis but not enough insulin to prevent hyperglycemia. In IDDM, hyperglycemia and ketoacidosis both occur.

  The nursing care for NIDDM is the same as for IDDM except the client may be given oral hypoglycemics instead of insulin. The client usually needs to be encouraged to lose weight.

A couple of days after Mr. Phillips has been diagnosed with DM he said to the nurse, "One of my friends at work said there are a lot of future problems with diabetes. I am concerned about this. What are some of the problems? What can I do not to have these problems?"

- What would be appropriate responses of the nurse?

  Diabetes has complications like any other disease. Some possible complications are eye problems, renal disease, heart disease, and decreased circulation and feeling in the extremities. Many of these complications can be controlled by maintaining a balance between exercise, diet, and insulin. For these reasons, it is important for a diabetic to follow the prescribed treatment regimen.

Diabetes Mellitus

Pathophysiology	
Diagnostic Studies	
Signs and Symptoms	
Nursing Interventions	

TABLE 1   Grid of pathophysiology, diagnostic studies, signs and symptoms, and nursing interventions for diabetes mellitus.

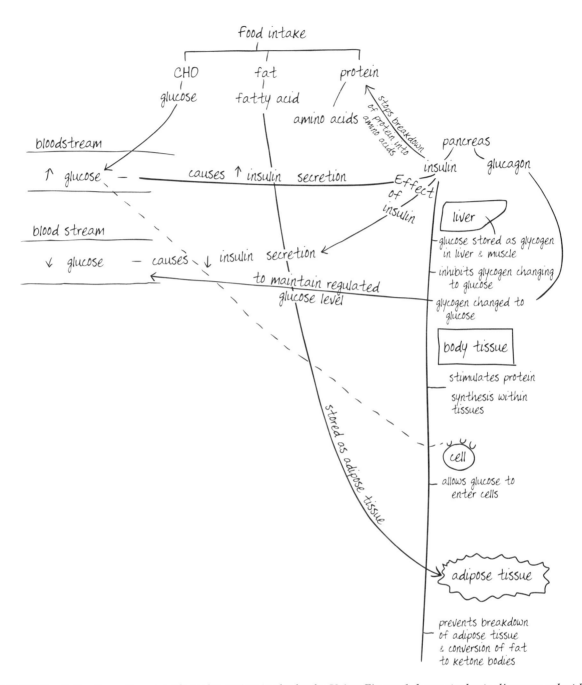

FIGURE 2 Patho-flow diagram of insulin action in the body. *Using Figure 1, have students diagram what happens in the body when insulin is not produced in adequate amounts or utilized appropriately.*

- What resources or support groups could Mr. Phillips be referred to in this locale?
  Resources and support groups are specific to each locale. Many local hospitals provide diabetic classes and/or support groups. Other resources are the American Diabetes Association and the National Diabetes Information Clearinghouse.
  The discharge teaching included insulin administration, diet, exercise, foot care, and eye exams.

- What is important to include in the discharge teaching regarding:
    insulin administration
  Teach Mr. Phillips the correct way to administer insulin, including the correct dose, time, and site.
  Teach Mr. Phillips that insulin is stored in a cool environment.
  Teach Mr. Phillips symptoms of hypoglycemia and hyperglycemia.

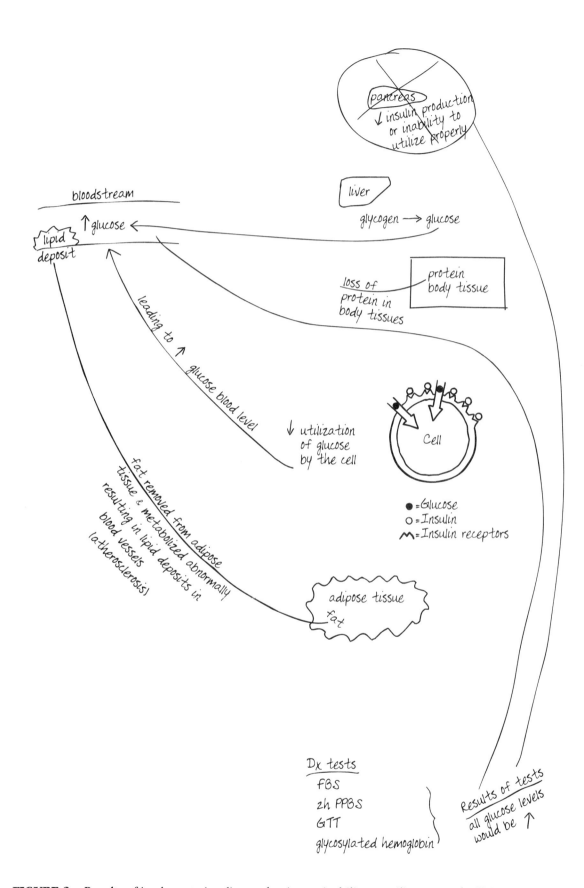

FIGURE 3   Results of inadequate insulin production or inability to utilize properly. *Using Figure 2, Patho-flow Diagram of Insulin Action in the Body, have students diagram what happens in the body when insulin is not produced in adequate amounts or not utilized appropriately.*

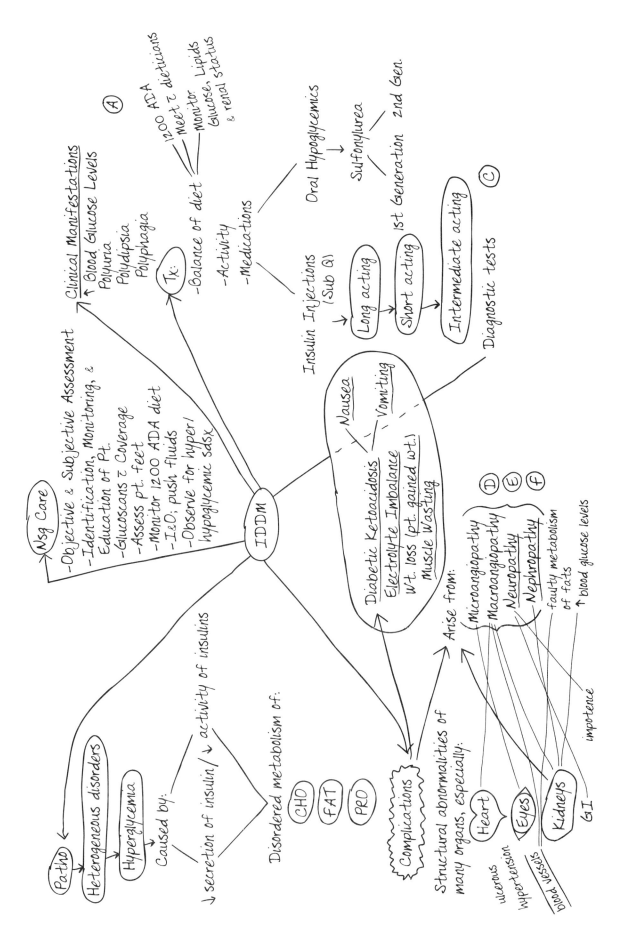

FIGURE 4 Concept Map of IDDM. Courtesy of Davette Kessel.

IDDM CONCEPT MAP

Patho   Nursing Care   Clinical Manifestations Ⓐ

Hyperglycemia

Caused by

Disordered metabolism of: IDDM

Carbohydrates   Treatment

Fat

Protein   Medications

                                                                  Insulin Injections; Oral Hypoglycemics

Complications   Common complications

Structural abnormalities   Arise from: Diagnostic Tests Ⓒ
of many organs, especially

Heart   Microangiopathy
                                      Macroangiopathy   Ⓓ
Eyes   Neuropathy   Ⓔ
                                      Nephropathy   Ⓕ
Kidneys

Gastrointestinal tract

Penis (impotence)

Blood vessels

A. Place a red asterisk (*) by all the symptoms Mr. Phillips may have been experiencing on admission.
B. Relate Mr. Phillip's symptoms to the etiological cause on the patho-flow chart by drawing a red line
    from the symptom to the etiological cause.
C. Write diagnostic tests the physician could use to confirm the diagnosis of diabetes mellitus. Draw a blue
    line to indicate the etiology for the results of the diagnostic tests. This may be easier to do on Figure 3.
D. Match the renal complications with the etiological cause.
E. Indicate organs affected by sensiomotor neuropathy.
F. Indicate organs affected by autonomic neuropathy.

FIGURE 5 Concept map of insulin dependent diabetes mellitus (IDDM). Courtesy of Davette Kessel.

diet
Refer the client to a nutritionist for client-specific diabetic instructions.
Eat meals and snacks at consistent times each day to interact with prescribed medications.
Alcohol may increase the risk of hypoglycemic reactions for clients on insulin or sulfonylureas.
exercise
Maintain a regular exercise program.
**Diabetics are not to exercise at the time of peak insulin action, when glucose is more than 250
mg/dL, or if ketones are present in the urine.**
foot care
Refer to Table 30-9 on page 842 in the core textbook.

eye exams
Have regular yearly eye exams.
If visual disturbances, such as blurred vision occur, notify the physician.

- Develop a care plan for Mr. Phillips.
Many nursing care plan examples are given in the core textbook. Refer to the diabetic client sample nursing care plan on pages 843–845 in the core textbook. Students are encouraged to include nursing diagnoses, goals, nursing interventions, rationale, and evaluation in their nursing care plans.

Eight years after Mr. Phillips was diagnosed with DM, he had a routine physical exam. At that time his BP was 174/96. The physician monitored the BP for three weeks and then placed Mr. Phillips on enalapril maleate (Vasotec). His urine had a trace of albumin.

- Physiologically what could be occurring to cause Mr. Phillips to have hypertension, which is a common complication of diabetes?
Sometimes diabetics do not metabolize lipids correctly and lipids adhere to blood vessel walls, causing the development of atherosclerosis. When plaque builds in the vessels, more pressure is needed to pump the blood through the vessels, resulting in hypertension.

- How does the action of enalapril maleate (Vasotec) lower the blood pressure?
Vasotec blocks the production of angiotension II, a potent vasodilator, which results in systemic vasodilation. By causing all vessels to dilate, pressure within the vessels is decreased and the blood pressure decreases.

- What is the rationale for placing Mr. Phillips on enalapril maleate (Vasotec) rather than propranolol (Inderal), verapamil (Calan), or clonidine (Catapres)?
Vasotec, an ACE inhibitor, blocks the production of angiotension II. ACE inhibitors are especially good for diabetics because they reduce proteinuria and slow the progress of nephropathy. Inderal is a beta blocker. Beta blockers cause a diabetic to become hypoglycemic and block the symptoms of hypoglycemia by blocking the sympathetic nervous system. Beta blockers also block gluconeogenesis and glycogenolysis, which are the body's natural ways of handling hypoglycemia. Calan is a calcium channel blocker, which inhibits calcium from moving into the vascular smooth muscle and causing contraction or vasoconstriction. Catapres acts on the central nervous center, inhibiting vasoconstriction.

- What other complications could have a circulatory etiology?

retinopathy	**myocardial infarction**
nephropathy	**cerebral vascular disease**
macrovascular disease	**cerebral vascular accident**
coronary artery disease	**peripheral vascular disease (PVD)**
angina	**extremity amputation**

- What could be the possible long-term renal complication from diabetes mellitus?
Diabetic nephropathy develops into chronic renal failure.

- Explain the pathophysiology of renal complications as they relate to DM. Relate these to the patho-flow diagram previously developed.
In diabetics, glomerular changes occur, causing decreased glomerulus filtration. The afferent and efferent blood vessels also become arteriosclerotic. The first sign of renal damage is protein in the urine, which is indicative of increased glomerular capillary permeability. Also refer to Figure 4.

One evening, Mr. Phillips was massaging his foot while watching television. He noticed an ulcerated area between his third and fourth toe.

- State possible reasons Mr. Phillips may not have felt pain from the ulcerated area. Relate these to the patho-flow diagram previously developed.
Diabetic neuropathy causes two types of neuropathies, sensorimotor polyneuropathy (peripheral neuropathy) and autonomic neuropathy. Peripheral neuropathy causes paresthesia and decreased pain and temperature sensations. Also refer to Figure 4.

During a yearly physical Mr. Phillips relates difficulty obtaining an erection.

- Explain the rationale for this complication.
Autonomic neuropathy may cause some diabetics to develop impotence.

- What nursing interventions would be appropriate at this time?
  Explain pathophysiology for difficulty obtaining an erection.
  Explain tests to check for impotence.
  Explain other options to satisfy sexual desires or obtain an erection.
  Encourage Mr. Phillips to tell the physician he is having sexual dysfunction.

  In later years, Mr. Phillips may experience some symptoms from autonomic neuropathies.

- List symptoms that may occur and relate the symptoms to the pathophysiological etiology.
  Gastrointestinal—delayed gastric emptying, constipation, diarrhea
  Urinary—urinary retention, neurogenic bladder, chronic renal failure
  Sexual dysfunction

CRITICAL THINKING EXERCISE WITH CIRRHOSIS

Sam Lightfoot, a sixty-year-old male of Native American descent, was admitted to the hospital with hematemesis. He has a history of alcohol abuse. Sam's wife and two daughters accompany him. Sam is 5′ 10″ tall and weighs 140 lbs. His vital signs are T 98.2, AP 98 and slightly irregular, R 24, BP 152/88. He is lethargic, confused, and jaundiced. When the nurse assessed his lung sounds, she heard pulmonary crackles in all lobes. His abdominal girth measures 44 inches. His wife states he has not gone to the bathroom all morning. He has +3 edema in his feet and ankles. Sam's primary diagnosis is hematemesis with a secondary diagnosis of cirrhosis.

- Brainstorm other subjective and objective data that are important to include in the assessment of Sam Lightfoot.

Subjective:	**history of hematemesis—how long has he had it, how often, amount, relationship to diet/alcohol**
	fatigue
	anorexia
	weakness
	indigestion
	difficulty breathing
	weight gain/loss
Objective:	**enlargement of liver and spleen**
	petechiae
	fever
	epistaxis
	breath sounds

- Relate the pathophysiology of cirrhosis to the assessed symptoms and other symptoms Sam may have experienced. Develop a patho-flow chart relating the symptoms to the pathological cause.
  Refer to Figure 6 for an example of a patho-flow chart relating the symptoms to the pathological cause.

- List diagnostic tests that would be appropriate for the physician to order for Sam. What abnormal laboratory results would be typical of cirrhosis?

CBC	**low WBCs, RBCs, Hgb, and platelets**
bilirubin	**elevated**
alkaline phosphatase	**elevated**
GGT	**elevated**
ALT	**elevated**
AST	**elevated**
albumin	**low**
PT	**delayed**
PTT	**delayed**
clotting times	**delayed**

- Relate the possible results of the diagnostic tests to the developed patho-flow chart.
  Refer to Figure 6. Information in parentheses is diagnostic test results as they relate to the patho-flow chart.

- Besides alcohol abuse what are some other causes of cirrhosis?

  chronic hepatitis   **cancer**
  hemachromatosis   **sclerosing cholangitis**
  exposure to toxic substances

- List complications of cirrhosis caused by chronic alcohol abuse.

  malnutrition   **portal hypertension**
  hypoglycemia   **ascites**
  clotting disorders   **hepatic encephalopathy**
  jaundice   **hepatorenal syndrome leading to possible renal failure**

- Explain the pathophysiology of portal hypertension as it relates to cirrhosis. Relate these to the patho-flow chart previously developed.

  When the portal vein becomes obstructed because of liver disease, the vessels draining into the portal system become engorged. Some of these vessels are the esophageal, gastric, mesenteric, and splenic veins. Congestion of the esophageal vein causes esophageal varices. Distention of the rectal vein causes hemorrhoids and distension of the splenic vein results in splenomegaly. Fluid also accumulates in the peritoneal cavity, resulting in ascites (refer to the patho-flow chart in Figure 6).

- List diuretics that may be ordered for Sam to decrease the ascites.

  spironolactone (Aldactone)
  Other potassium-sparing diuretics are amiloride (Midamor) and triamterene (Dyrenium).

- How does the action of lactulose (Cephulac) lower the level of ammonia in the blood?

  Ammonia moves from the blood into the bowel. Lactulose acts as a laxative and excretes stool containing ammonia.

- What other complications result from portal hypertension?

  esophageal varices   **splenomegaly**
  hemorrhoids   **pleural effusion**

- Explain the rationale for the complication of pleural effusion.

  As the venous system becomes congested, fluid starts accumulating in the lungs, causing pleural effusion.

- Identify possible nursing diagnoses for Sam.

  Thought processes, altered, related to elevated serum ammonia level and hepatic coma
  Fluid volume, excess, related to ascites
  Skin integrity, impaired, high risk for, related to accumulation of bile salts in skin, poor skin turgor, ascites, and edema
  Nutrition, altered, less than body requirements related to inadequate diet, anorexia, or vomiting
  (Refer to the possible nursing diagnoses for cirrhosis on page 998 in the core textbook.)

- What nursing interventions would be appropriate at this time?

  Monitor confusion and lethargy.
  Elevate bedrails to prevent injury.
  Monitor laboratory reports for ammonia level.
  Provide low-protein diet.
  Weigh daily.
  Measure abdominal girth daily.
  Monitor fluid restriction as ordered.
  Provide egg crate mattress.
  Turn client every two hours.
  Apply lotion to skin frequently, especially to pressure areas.
  Provide low-sodium diet as ordered.
  Offer frequent small, high-calorie meals and/or high nutrient supplements as ordered.
  Provide frequent oral hygiene.

- Develop a care plan for Sam Lightfoot.

  Refer to the possible nursing diagnoses for a cirrhosis client on page 998 in the textbook. It is important that the student's care plan be individualized for Sam Lightfoot.

Symptoms of Cirrhosis
  hematemesis
  fatigue
  anorexia
  indigestion
  difficulty breathing
  pulmonary congestion
  weight gain/loss
  enlarged liver
  enlarged spleen
  fever
  epitaxis
  elevated AP
  elevated systolic BP
  lethargic
  confused
  jaundice
  ascites
  edema

The damaged liver can
not filter blood and
destroy bacteria present.

↓

fever

Degenerative changes occur ⟵ (Enzymes in the liver are alkaline
in liver tissues   phosphatase, GGT, ALT, and AST.
↓   A damaged liver results in elevated
Enlarged liver   levels of these enzymes.)
↓
Blood flowing into the portal
vein cannot flow through the
liver because the liver is
damaged (portal hypertension).
Blood vessels flowing into the
portal vein become congested.

↓

As blood accumulates ⎫   esophageal varices ⟶ esophageal vessels ⟶ Congested esophageal veins
in the vessels draining │   spleenomegaly   rupture   cause esophageal varices
into the portal vein,   ⎬ ⟶ ascites
plasma filtrates into   │   edema   ↓
the peritoneal cavity   ⎭   indigestion ⎫   hematemesis   Excess fluid in the abdomen
                              anorexia   ⎰ ⟵────────────────────────── slows digestion and decreases
                                                                         appetite
Malnutrition may be cause
for low WCBs, RBCs, and Hgb. ⟶

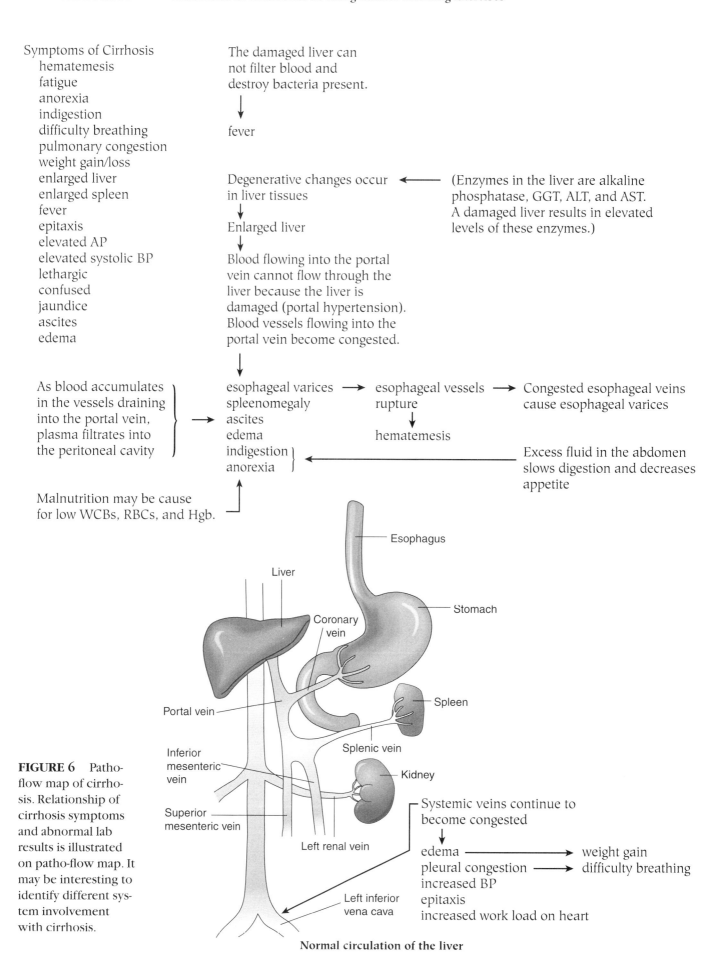

FIGURE 6 Patho-flow map of cirrhosis. Relationship of cirrhosis symptoms and abnormal lab results is illustrated on patho-flow map. It may be interesting to identify different system involvement with cirrhosis.

Esophagus
Liver
Coronary vein
Stomach
Spleen
Portal vein
Splenic vein
Inferior mesenteric vein
Kidney
Superior mesenteric vein
Left renal vein
Left inferior vena cava

Systemic veins continue to
become congested
↓
edema ⟶ weight gain
pleural congestion ⟶ difficulty breathing
increased BP
epitaxis
increased work load on heart

Normal circulation of the liver

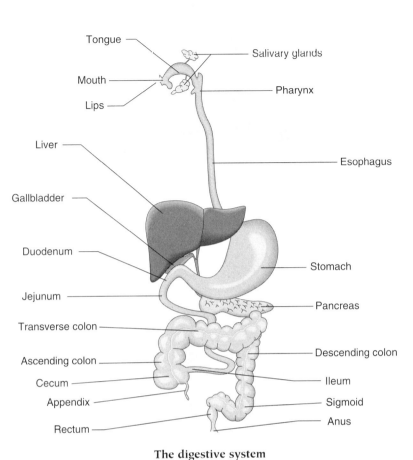

Liver is unable to filter ◄───── (low albumin)
proteins and protein
byproducts

↓

ammonia accumulates in ─────┐
bloodstream   │

↓   │

hepatic encephalopathy   │

↓   │

confusion   │
lethargy   │

toxins accumulate in body ◄─┘

↑

liver unable to detoxify toxins

The damaged liver is
unable to produce
prothrombin and
fibrinogen which are
needed for clotting.

↓

(delayed PT, PTT,
and clotting time)

The digestive system

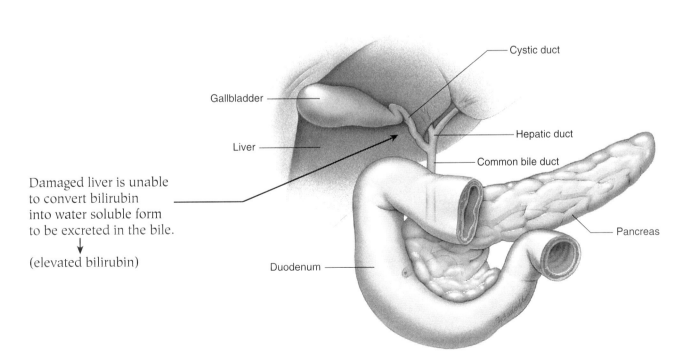

Damaged liver is unable
to convert bilirubin
into water soluble form
to be excreted in the bile.

↓

(elevated bilirubin)

The biliary tree

Cirrhosis

Pathophysiology	
Diagnostic Studies	
Signs and Symptoms	
Nursing Interventions	

Table 2   Grid of pathophysiology, diagnostic studies, signs and symptoms, and nursing interventions for cirrhosis.

- If Sam's condition improved and he was scheduled for discharge, what is important to include in the discharge teaching regarding:

    bleeding tendencies

    Follow through with scheduled lab tests. Explain to Sam that he could bleed and bruise easily, therefore, he should be cautious and/or avoid situations when he could be injured.

    exercise

    Fatigue is a common symptom of cirrhosis, therefore, balance activity with rest periods.

    weight gain

    Weigh self regularly. Notify physician of weight gain of 1½ pounds or more in one week.
    Teach client how to measure correct amount of fluids.
    Refer to dietitian for sodium restricted diet.

    skin care

    Closely monitor skin for redness or broken skin in edematous areas.
    Apply lotion to skin and edematous areas.

- Explain diet instructions for Sam Lightfoot. Consider cultural influence in the diet instructions.

    Sodium may be restricted to 2 grams or less per day. Have Sam and his wife list foods eaten on a regular basis. Calculate sodium intake according to foods he eats.

    Sam is to avoid alcoholic beverages. Share the names of beverages that are not alcoholic that could be substituted for alcoholic beverages.

- List local resources/support groups where Sam and his family could be referred.

    Alcoholics Anonymous is one resource group where Sam and his family could be referred. Each locale will have other resources available.

Sam's daughter, Mary, says, "I wish Dad would have quit drinking years ago. I was always embarrassed by his behavior when he had too much to drink. His life could have had so much potential."

- What would be appropriate responses of the nurse?

    Some responses could be:

    Your father caused you much embarrassment.

    Living with an alcoholic is often difficult. His drinking often embarrassed you because his actions were inappropriate.

    His drinking prevented him from reaching his potential and caused you much embarrassment.

Encourage students to share how they would respond. Discuss the responses shared. Perhaps role playing may be helpful to increase communication skills.

CRITICAL THINKING EXERCISE WITH HYPERTENSION, CONGESTIVE HEART FAILURE, AND CHRONIC RENAL FAILURE

Trina Brown, a forty-year-old African American female, has had hypertension for twenty years. She has been non-compliant in taking her antihypertensive medications that were prescribed by her physician. She has recently developed symptoms of congestive heart failure and renal failure.

- Brainstorm some reasons for Trina's noncompliance.

    Some possible reasons for Trina's noncompliance are finances, lack of knowledge of disease process and future complications, lack of transportation, feels "good" and does not see reason for medication, and does not like side effects of medications. Students may list others also.

- Name some medications that may have been prescribed to treat Trina's hypertension. List the advantage and disadvantage of each medication.

    Table 3 may be helpful for the students in completing this exercise. Table 5 is an adaptation of Table 21-1 on page 510 in the core textbook. Refer to Table 4 for medications that may be prescribed and the advantages and disadvantages of each medication.

Hypertension, Congestive Heart Failure, and Chronic Renal Failure

Pathophysiology	
Diagnostic Studies	
Signs and Symptoms	
Nursing Interventions	

Table 3   Grid of pathophysiology, diagnostic studies, signs and symptoms, and nursing interventions for hypertension, congestive heart failure, and chronic renal failure.

Antihypertensive Medications	Advantages	Disadvantages
Alpha-adrenergic Blockers clonidine hydrochloride (Catapres) doxazosin mesylate (Cardura) methyldopa (Aldomet) phentolamine mesylate (Regitine) prazosin hydrochloride (Minipress) terazosin hydrochloride (Vasocard, Hytrin)		
Angiotensin-converting Enzyme (ACE) Inhibitors captopril (Capoten) enalapril maleate (Vasotec)		
Calcium Channel Blockers diltiazem hydrochloride (Cardizem) nifedipine (Procardia) verapamil (Calan, Isoptin)		
Ganglionic Blocker trimethaphan camsylate (Arfonad)		
Loop Diuretics bumetanide (Bumex) furosemide (Lasix)		
Potassium-sparing Diuretics amiloride hydrochloride (Midamor) spironolactone (Aldactone) spironolactone with HCTZ (Aldactazide) triamterene (Dyrenium)		

(continued)

Antihypertensive Medications	Advantages	Disadvantages
Thiazide Diuretics chlorothiazide (Diuril) hydrochlorothiazide (Esdrix, HydroDIURIL) methyclothiazide (Enduron) metolazone (Zaroxolyn)		
Thiazide-like Diuretics chlorthalidone (Hygroton) indapamide (Lozol)		
Peripherally Acting Adrenergic Antagonists reserpine (Serpasil)		
Direct-acting Vasodilators daizoxide (Hyperstat) hydralazine hydrochloride (Apresoline) nitroprusside sodium (Nipride)		

TABLE 4   Antihypertensive Medications

- Using Table 35-2, Chronic Renal Failure Effects on Body Systems, develop a concept map showing the relationship of hypertension to the effects of renal failure on each listed system.
  Since several examples have been given in the text and in the instructor's guide, now is the time for the students to have an opportunity to develop their own concept map. Have fun and be creative!

- What is the relationship between hypertension, increased peripheral resistance, cardiac hypertrophy, and congestive heart failure?
  Disease processes, such as arteriosclerosis and atherosclerosis, cause vessels to lose elasticity, resulting in increased peripheral resistance. If blood vessels are unable to expand or contract, pressure increases in the vessels, resulting in hypertension. If vessels have increased peripheral resistance, more force is needed to pump the blood through the body. This causes a heavier workload on the heart, which causes cardiac hypertrophy. If the heart has an increased workload for an extended period, it is finally not able to meet the demands of the body, resulting in CHF.

- What is the relationship between blood pressure (hypotension and hypertension) and renal failure?
  Prolonged hypertension causes the elastic tissue in blood vessels to be replaced with a fibrous collagen tissue that is not able to expand and contract. This leads to increased peripheral resistance and decreased blood flow to vital organs such as the brain, heart, and kidneys. When the blood flow to the kidneys is decreased, the vessels in the kidney constrict, causing renal ischemia. Prolonged renal ischemia causes renal tubular necrosis and renal failure.
  A systolic blood pressure of 70 or greater is needed to sustain adequate blood flow to the kidneys. If the systolic blood pressure drops below 70, renal failure occurs because the kidney vessels constrict, causing renal ischemia, renal tubular necrosis, and finally renal failure.

Antihypertensive Medications	Advantages	Disadvantages
Alpha-adrenergic Blockers clonidine hydrochloride (Catapres) doxazosin mesylate (Cardura) methyldopa (Aldomet) phentolamine mesylate (Regitine) prazosin hydrochloride (Minipress) terazosin hydrochloride (Vasocard, Hytrin)	These medications are an option for clients who cannot tolerate diuretics or beta blockers.	Some clients experience a first-dose phenomenon which is faintness, dizziness, or palpitation one to three hours after the initial dose. If Catapres and Aldomet are taken over a long period they may cause sodium and fluid retention, causing hypertension. Catapres may cause rebound hypertension if medication is stopped abruptly. If Catapres is discontinued, the dosage should be tapered off slowly over seven days.
Angiotensin-converting Enzyme (ACE) Inhibitors captopril (Capoten) enalapril maleate (Vasotec)	Work well for diabetic clients. Do not affect respiratory system like beta blockers. Do not raise uric acid levels. Do not lower potassium levels.	African-Americans sometimes may have to take a diuretic along with these medications. Have a side effect of angioedema of the face, extremities, lips, tongue, glottis, and larynx. Some clients develop a chronic cough.
Calcium Channel Blockers diltiazem hydrochloride (Cardizem) nifedipine (Procardia) verapamil (Calan, Isoptin)	Recommended for clients who can not tolerate or have not found diuretics and beta blockers to work well. Safer to use in patients with diabetes, gout, and hyperlipidemia.	Cardizem and Calan may cause heart failure in clients with ventricular dysfunction.
Ganglionic Blocker trimethaphan camsylate (Arfonad)		
Loop Diuretics bumetanide (Bumex) furosemide (Lasix)	Start working faster than thiazides and may be good for clients with renal problems and congestive heart failure.	Less effective for hypertension than thiazides. Deplete the body of potassium.
Potassium-sparing Diuretics amiloride hydrochloride (Midamor) spironolactone (Aldactone) spironolactone with HCTZ (Aldactazide) triamterene (Dyrenium)	Does not deplete the body of potassium like other diuretics.	Monitor for hyperkalemia especially in clients with diabetes and/or renal problems.

(continued)

Antihypertensive Medications	Advantages	Disadvantages
Thiazide Diuretics chlorothiazide (Diuril) hydrochlorothiazide (Esdrix, HydroDIURIL) methyclothiazide (Enduron) metolazone (Zaroxolyn)	Inexpensive Easy to administer African-Americans respond well to these diuretics.	Takes several days for medication to start working and up to four weeks before medication reaches full therapeutic level. Monitor potassium level. Diabetics may have glucose intolerance when taking these medications.
Thiazide-like Diuretics chlorthalidone (Hygroton) indapamide (Lozol)	Inexpensive Easy to administer. Work well in African-Americans.	May cause glucose intolerance and hypokalemia.
Peripherally Acting Adrenergic Antagonists reserpine (Serpasil)		Postural hypotension is a side effect.
Direct-acting Vasodilators daizoxide (Hyperstat) hydralazine hydrochloride (Apresoline) nitroprusside sodium (Nipride)		Monitor for tachycardia which can cause angina pectoris in clients with coronary artery disease.

TABLE 5   Antihypertensive Medications

- What is the relationship between the heart's decreasing ability to pump blood through the blood vessels and pulmonary edema?
  When the heart is unable to pump blood effectively through the body, blood backs up in the veins and the lungs fill with fluid. It is similar to the example of a dammed river. If the dam is closed and water keeps flowing into the river from melting snow or rain, the river will eventually fill and spill over the riverbank. The heart is the dam because it cannot pump effectively and keeps blood backed up behind the heart. Eventually the blood fills the lungs and causes congestion/edema.

- Explain the relationship between fluid in the alveoli and dyspnea.
  Alveoli are surrounded with capillaries in which oxygen and carbon dioxide are exchanged between the alveoli and capillaries. If the alveoli are filled with fluid, there is less space for the exchange of oxygen and carbon dioxide. Refer to Figure 19-1 on page 389 and Figure 19-3 on page 392 in the core textbook.

- Physiologically, what is occurring in Trina's body to cause an increased rate of respiration?
  In congestive heart failure, the heart is unable to pump blood effectively through the body so there is not an internal exchange of oxygen and carbon dioxide (internal respiration). The carbon dioxide level increases in the body and the respiratory center stimulates respirations to increase. The lungs are congested and there is not an adequate exchange of oxygen and carbon dioxide (external respiration). Because of symptoms of renal failure, toxins are accumulating in Trina's body and her respirations are increasing to rid the body of the toxins.

- List laboratory results that would indicate that Trina is developing chronic renal failure.
  BUN more than 50, Creatine more than 3

- List symptoms that would indicate Trina is developing chronic renal failure.
  nocturia and polyuria

- List subjective and objective data for which the nurse would assess for symptoms of chronic renal failure.

  Subjective: **fatigue**
  joint pain
  headaches
  nausea
  anorexia
  hiccups
  impaired concentration
  decreased libido
  menstrual irregularities
  Objective: **halitosis with urine odor**
  increased respirations which develop into Kussmaul respirations as condition progresses

- List laboratory results that would indicate that Trina is developing congestive heart failure.
  chest x-ray—enlargement of left ventricle and lung congestion, EKG

- List symptoms that would indicate Trina is developing congestive heart failure.

cyanosis	**low BP**	**fatigue**
tachycardia	**restless**	**decreased urinary output**
dyspneic		

- List subjective and objective data for which the nurse would assess for symptoms of congestive heart failure.

  Subjective: **dyspnea**
  orthopnea
  fatigue
  anxiety
  chest pain
  difficulty performing ADLs
  Objective: **LOC**
  skin for cyanosis or pallor
  skin turgor
  jugular distention
  breath sounds or adventitious sounds
  normal/abnormal S_1 and S_2 sounds
  check for S_3 sounds
  hypoactive bowel sounds
  quality of peripheral pulses
  capillary refill
  edema—extremities and abdomen
  weight gains/losses
  monitor I&O for oliguria

- Identify possible nursing diagnoses for Trina.

- List nursing interventions and give rationale for each intervention.
  Refer to the following core textbook examples of nursing diagnoses and nursing interventions for Trina:

  1. **Possible nursing diagnoses for a client with congestive heart failure on page 484.**
  2. **Sample Nursing Care Plan: The Client with Hypertension on page 512.**
  3. **Possible nursing diagnoses for a client with end stage renal disease (ESRD) on page 1046.**

Trina's abdomen is distended and she has lost her appetite for the last two days. She has had hiccups constantly for two hours. She says, "I am so tired of these hiccups. Why am I having them?"

- Explain to Trina the cause for her hiccups.
  Uremia is thought to cause CNS stimulation of the phrenic nerve. Irritation of the phrenic nerve causes intermittent spasming of the diaphragm, which is the cause of hiccups. Acid-base and electrolyte imbalances may also cause hiccups.

REFERENCES/SUGGESTED READINGS

Chase, S. (1997). Antihypertensives. *RN, 97(6)*, 33–39.

CHAPTER 1
Introduction to Critical Thinking

This chapter is designed to introduce students to the process of critical thinking by explaining the basic concepts in easy-to-understand language. It also introduces the student to the textbook itself by explaining its basic features, such as key terms, learning objectives, key abbreviations, review questions, sample care plans, and case studies. It provides the student with tips on how to best utilize these elements. It is suggested that you spend some time exploring this chapter with your students in order to lay a solid foundation of study.

The following sections have been extracted from Chapter 1:

LEARNING OBJECTIVES

Upon completion of this chapter, the learner should be able to:

1. Explain the relationship between critical thinking and the nursing process.
2. State five characteristics of the person who uses critical thinking.
3. Identify behaviors which illustrate the traits of a nurse who is a critical thinker.
4. Assess own strengths and weaknesses in relation to critical thinking skills.
5. Develop a personal plan for the enhancement of personal critical thinking and reasoning skills.

SUMMARY

- Critical thinking is a disciplined way of thinking that the nursing student can begin to develop. The effective use of the nursing process depends on the ability to think well.
- There are many ways to define critical thinking, but an exact definition does not lead anyone to become a good thinker. Essential components of any definition should emphasize that critical thinking is concerned with self-assessment of the quality of one's own thinking, according to standards of excellence and careful use of the elements of reasoning.
- There are four basic intellectual skills that are essential to quality thinking. These skills are critical reading, critical writing, critical listening, and critical speaking.
- The Spectrum of Universal Intellectual Standards can be the measure of competence in each of the basic skills.
- Reasoning is the process of applying critical thinking to some problem to find an answer or to figure something out. Therefore, reasoning has a purpose. The process of reasoning requires that attention be paid to the elements of thought in reasoning and to the universal intellectual standards.
- When students begin to be aware of their own thinking and begin to assume responsibility for it, they will begin to use their own logic to discover the logic of nursing. The result will be better learning and the ability to use the nursing process to make high-quality decisions related to client care.
- Consistent attention to improving the quality of thinking will produce the traits of an educated nurse. The student will become intellectually reasonable, humble, courageous, and possess intellectual integrity and perseverance.

CASE STUDY

At this point in subsequent chapters you will be given a client scenario or case study. This activity is designed to give you an opportunity to apply the knowledge and skills you have gained. This will mean that you will be expected to use critical thinking skills to apply the nursing process as you explore selected nursing situations.

For this chapter the scenario is to be written by you and about you. In order to do this, you will use the nursing process to develop your plan for improving and utilizing your reasoning and thinking skills. This is a suggested way for you to approach this exercise.

1. Review the four basic skills for critical thinking: reading, writing, listening, and speaking.
2. Utilize the nursing process step of assessment to assess your skills in each area. Assessment implies that you will use the standards for skill in each of these areas to identify your own strengths and weaknesses.
3. Identify specifically the precise skills you want to improve. Write in your own words what you want to accomplish in terms of positive skills you will possess when you have implemented your plan and accomplished your goal. This means that you will identify specific performance measures for your reading, writing, speaking, and listening skills and time frames for points at which you will evaluate your performance. For example, if you set a goal of being able to identify the main points of assigned reading, how would you measure that? By comparison with others in your study group? By your test performance? Write down your evaluation criteria and the time for evaluation. This step corresponds to the nursing process steps of diagnosis and goal setting.
4. When you have clearly stated in writing which basic skills you will work on, you are ready to move to the next step of the nursing process, which is planning. Review the material in this chapter or from other resources to identify possible ways to work on your skills. Choose the most appropriate methods for you. Write down your plan. Be precise and specific.
5. Your next step, as in the nursing process, is to actually put your plan in action by doing what you have planned to do. This is the implementation step.
6. The final step of the nursing process is evaluation. This simply means look to see if your actions have resulted in the desired outcome. In order to perform a valid evaluation, you must have something with which to measure. In the case of nursing process in client care, evaluation is based on the goals which were set during the problem identification and goal-setting steps. When the time for evaluation arrives, you make a judgment about how well your goal has been met. If the goal is met, reassess for the next area needing work and start over. If your goal is not met to your satisfaction, repeat the process.
7. Realize that you must know yourself well. If the processes of critical thinking and reasoning are new to you, select only one or two things to work on. If you feel more adventurous, use the suggested process to explore your thinking in relation to the universal standards of thought and to the traits of a thoughtful person. Assess your problem-solving style in relation to the elements of thought in reasoning.

REVIEW QUESTIONS

This section in the following chapters will have a set of NCLEX style review questions. It will be important for you to understand that these questions provide an opportunity for you to practice your growing critical thinking skills. It is tempting to use review questions simply as a way to collect an isolated fact—the "correct" answer to this question. To improve your test-taking skills, look at each question as an opportunity to apply reasoning skills. To illustrate this, let's look at a possible thought pattern applied to a sample question.

Do not be concerned if you do not know the answer to this sample question. It has been selected deliberately to represent some knowledge you will probably be presented later in the course so that you will not guess or try to choose the answer intuitively. Focus on the thought processes illustrated.

Question: What is the most basic assessment to make about a client receiving IV potassium?
> a. hourly urine output
> b. vital signs
> c. neuromuscular status
> d. EKG recordings

This is an example of an approach to answering this question using the elements of thought in reasoning:

1. What is the purpose of this question? Why did the instructor choose this question?
    Possible answer: To test how well I understand the nursing implications for the IV administration of potassium.

2. State the problem to be solved. What is the question at issue?
    Possible answer: The question asks me to identify the most basic assessment to make when a client is receiving IV potassium. The key here is to identify the basic assessment which an LP/VN would be expected to make.

3. Read all of the possible answers in light of the question at issue. Apply the process of reasoning to each of them. Remember, it is as important to know why an answer is wrong for this question as to know why an answer is right. Let's look at each possible response.

a. hourly urine output

This may be a good choice because it is an assessment that you as an LP/VN will be prepared to make. Your knowledge base will also have provided the information that potassium is a vital electrolyte that is excreted by the kidney. You will also have learned that it can accumulate in the serum when urine output is decreased. This accumulation can lead to the adverse effects of too much potassium. At this point, you will consider this a good candidate for the right answer, but you will want to consider the other options as well.

b. vital signs

This looks good. Most students consider assessment of vital signs a good answer most of the time. Let's look at the evidence. Your knowledge base has included the information that a potassium deficit or excess can affect the blood pressure and the regularity of the heart beat. Before you select this answer, however, ask yourself when does this effect take place? When the levels are abnormal. What is the greatest danger of IV potassium? Too much potassium. But here is the key question: what is the most basic assessment to make for IV potassium? What can cause the potassium level to be too high in this situation? Decreased excretion of potassium, which comes from decreased urine output. So this answer is not best for this question. Assessing vital signs is important and should be done for this client, but it is not the most basic because it is a later indication of change and not specific for potassium.

c. neuromuscular status

As usual, this answer also looks good. Your knowledge base will have given you the information that changes in potassium level can affect muscle tone and reflexes. Review the question one more time: which of the possible answers is the most basic assessment in relation to IV potassium. Again, changes in neuromuscular status are important to assess, but these changes are indicators of a problem resulting from changes in the potassium level. Urine output is an indicator of the ability of the body to handle potassium. So you conclude that this is not the best answer to this question. This does not mean that it is not an important assessment for this client. The question at issue is what is the most basic assessment.

d. EKG recordings

Here is another attractive answer. You will probably learn that changes in potassium can affect the EKG (ECG) tracing and cause cardiac dysrhythmias. There are two reasons why this is not the best answer for this question. First, these changes are late and do not match well with the potassium level, so this is not the most basic assessment. Second, most LP/VN students are not expected to make this kind of interpretation of EKG's. This does not mean that this is not an important assessment. It is not the most basic for an LP/VN.

So, this process, which takes much longer for me to write and for you to read than it does to do, leads us to the conclusion that response (a) is correct. You can see that preparing for and answering the review questions will be much more interesting than simply trying to memorize some fact or to identify the correct answer by memory.

CHAPTER 2
Legal Aspects of Nursing

SUGGESTED RESPONSES TO CASE STUDY I

Case Study I: Helen Gee

Helen Gee is admitted for diabetes out of control. She is very nervous about this admission, despite the fact that she has been hospitalized several times before. Helen is unable to discuss advance directives with the social services representative at this time. "It makes me too nervous to think about that stuff," she explained to the social worker.

Later, Helen and two of her daughters were discussing a case they heard about on the news. A family had petitioned the court to disconnect a respirator on their daughter who had been in a persistent vegetative state for two years.

Helen said, "If I get bad, don't you kids pull the plug on me. I want you to do everything possible." Everyone laughed and the daughters made a couple of joking comments. The nurse joined in the discussion, asking pointed questions about Helen's beliefs regarding life-sustaining measures.

1. Was the nurse out of line to enter into a private discussion?
    The nurse was not out of line to enter into this private discussion. She had information to offer pertaining to the topic and there was data she needed to collect. This was an ideal time to do needed teaching about the concept of advance directives.

2. Does Helen's statement, "Don't pull the plug" qualify as an advance directive? List rationale.
    Helen's statement does qualify as an advance directive. She is giving information about what she wishes to happen to her in the future. It would be best to have this information in writing, but she is clearly indicating what she wants or does not want to happen.

3. List factors the nurse should emphasize when attempting to explain the concepts of advance directives.
    The nurse should emphasize the client's right to self-determination, and explain definitions of power of attorney, health care representative, living wills, and life-prolonging declarations.

    The client retains the right to make all health care decisions as long as he/she is of sound mind. Clients may change their minds about health care decisions at any time. Advance directives serve as a guide for family members and the physician. Advance directives are best given in writing and only go into effect should the individual have a terminal illness or when death is imminent.

4. Write a sample documentation of this interaction.
    Client and daughters discussing news story where family requested discontinuing life support on daughter in persistent vegetative state. Mrs. Gee stated, "Don't you kids pull the plug on me. I want you to do everything you can." Discussed concepts of advance directives, explaining living will, life-prolonging procedures declaration, durable power of attorney for health care, and health care representative. Encouraged client to consider putting her wishes in writing. Social services referral initiated.

SUGGESTED RESPONSES TO CASE STUDY II

Case Study II: Mr. Jones

Mr. Jones is admitted for congestive heart failure. He is sixty-six years old, newly diagnosed, and acutely ill at this time. A student LP/VN is assisting the registered nurse (RN) with the admission. The student notes that Mr. Jones has a living will. Later she asks the RN, "Will you have to contact the doctor regarding a No Code status for Mr. Jones? He's got a living will so he doesn't want anything done."

1. List factors the nurse should explain to assist the student in understanding the concept of the living will.
    The living will declaration explains that certain life-prolonging procedures not be used in the event that death is imminent. However, Mr. Jones is diagnosed with congestive heart failure, a treatable condition, from which he is expected to recover. The living will declaration would not apply unless his condition worsened significantly.

2. Describe how a cardiac arrest might impact this situation.
    A cardiac arrest could significantly alter Mr. Jones' prognosis. Should it become necessary to consider placing him on some form of life support, like a ventilator, then the living will declaration would become a factor.

    Mr. Jones' wife speaks privately with the nurse. She states, "I want everything possible done to save my husband. I don't care what it takes."

3. Describe how this information may or may not affect the living will requests that Mr. Jones has made.
    Mr. Jones has the right to determine the course of his health care. However, when the wishes of the family members conflict with the wishes of the terminal client, the health team find themselves in a quandary. The concern is that the bereaved will bring suit against the physician and

the facility. The advance directives serve as a guide, but may not be the deciding factor in a precarious situation.

4. Write how the nurse might respond in this situation.
    "Mrs. Jones, I understand your concern for your husband. However, let's reconsider what he would like to happen. He has expressed several times that he does not want to live hooked up to a machine. Would you want him to live like that? Let us discuss the options contained in the living will declaration so you have a clear understanding of what is involved."

5. Identify a nursing diagnosis, two goals, and expected outcomes for Mrs. Jones.
    Nursing Diagnosis: **Coping, ineffective, individual, related to husband's health care status.**
    Goal 1: **Mrs. Jones will identify fears regarding husband's health status.**
    Outcome: **Mrs. Jones will plan how to address her personal fears regarding her husband's health status.**
    Goal 2: **Mrs. Jones will verbalize basic concepts associated with client's right to self-determination.**
    Outcome: **Mrs. Jones will be more receptive to her husband's requests in the living declaration.**

    Mr. Jones is refusing a recommended treatment option. Mrs. Jones disagrees, and tells the doctor to go ahead with the recommended treatment plan.

6. How does the Patient Self-Determination Act affect Mr. Jones' refusal of treatment?
    Mr. Jones is competent, of sound mind, and responsible for his own health care decisions. According to the Patient Self-Determination Act, he has the right to refuse treatment, any treatment, even if not having that treatment means he may die.

7. List the parameters allowing Mrs. Jones to consent or refuse treatment for her husband.
    If Mr. Jones should become mentally incompetent and thus unable to make responsible decisions for his health care, then Mrs. Jones can give or deny consent for treatment.

    Bob Smith came to the hospital for outpatient diagnostic testing. Passing an open door, he saw his high school principal, Mr. Jones, lying in a bed. A respiratory therapist was giving Mr. Jones a treatment and there seemed to be tubes and bags hanging everywhere. Alarmed, Bob went to the nurse's station seeking information. He pointed to Mr. Jones' name and room number listed on the board, and began asking questions.

8. Discuss ways to calm Bob's fears without violating Mr. Jones' right to privacy.
    The nurse can assure Bob that the situation is not an emergency and that Mr. Jones is expected to make a full recovery; explain that much of the paraphernalia is routine, used for purposes of hydration or medication administration for many hospitalized clients; let Bob know that Mrs. Jones is sitting in the lounge and he can speak with her about the particulars of Mr. Jones' situation.

9. Identify what situation(s) have already occurred to violate this client's privacy.
    The door was open and the curtain was not pulled to shield the client from the view of people passing by the door while the respiratory treatment was administered.

ANSWERS TO THE REVIEW QUESTIONS

1. Standards of practice are:
    b. guidelines to direct nursing care.
2. Immunity for nurses giving care in emergency situations is provided under the:
    b. Good Samaritan Law.
3. Select the situation that violates client privacy:
    d. Talking about an interesting client in the cafeteria.
4. To make the best use of time in the clinical area, the nurse should:
    a. chart events as they happen.
5. The responsibility for informed consent rests with the:
    c. physician.
6. Informed consent occurs when the:
    c. client understands the risks, benefits, and alternatives to treatment.
7. If you suspect a co-worker is diverting drugs, you should:
    b. document dates, times, observed behavior, and report to your supervisor.

8. Advance directives:
   c. guide family members through difficult decisions.
9. The health care representative or durable power of attorney for health care:
   b. can give or withhold consent for treatment.
10. Which of the following situations reflects inappropriate use of an incident report?
    d. An instructor, frustrated with a disorganized student nurse, fills out an incident report because the student gave a 9 A.M. medication at 9:25.

CHAPTER 3
Introduction to Ethics

SUGGESTED RESPONSES TO CASE STUDY I

Janice is a forty-five-year-old woman who is pregnant with her fourth child. The pregnancy was unplanned and distressed Janice and her husband at first, but now they have accepted it and look forward to the delivery of their child. Janice has been receiving prenatal care from her family practice physician since her second month of pregnancy. She is now in her seventh month.

During her sixth month of pregnancy, the physician ordered laboratory tests and the results indicated a fetal abnormality. The physician requested to perform further invasive testing on the fetus during the seventh month. Janice and her husband refused further fetal testing. Although the physician explained the importance of the testing, the couple continued to refuse it.

After the couple leave the office the physician turns to the nurse and states, "Since they will not follow my suggestions, write them a letter and tell them I am terminating our relationship. Tell her to see a specialist." No arrangements for a referral have been made for Janice by the doctor. The doctor fears the high-risk delivery predisposes him to a lawsuit.

1. Based on the information presented here, what are the primary moral/ ethical issues?
   The parents may be concerned that, if an abnormality is found, the physician may recommend an abortion. The parents may be opposed to abortion and therefore are refusing fetal testing. The physician is angry that the parents are not following his requests and has terminated his services without following through with a referral. The physician may resent the parents not following his recommendations. The couple are coming from the concept that they have a right to choices in health care and desire to be a participant in their care. The physician is concerned that the parents may sue if complications arise in the pregnancy or during delivery. Because of his fears he has terminated his services without referral.

2. What are your personal values in relation to the situation?
   Each student must answer this individually based on personal values.

3. What course of action would you recommend for the nurse and why? What ethical/moral principles would guide you?
   The nurse could approach the doctor and ask him to reconsider talking to the couple after they have had time to adjust to the idea of an abnormality. The nurse could also request he provide a referral for the couple. The nurse is guided by a sense of responsibility for her clients.

4. To what extent, in your opinion, is Janice noncompliant?
   Answers will vary on this question. Possible responses may be:
   - **Janice is being compliant but is fearful of the end results of her pregnancy. She may be afraid**

the physician will suggest an abortion and she does not want to face the decision or may be opposed to that decision.
- **Janice is being noncompliant by not allowing the physician to do the tests.**

5. Was the medical intervention adequate? Is nursing to judge medical care?
Answers will vary. Some students say no because they think the physician should talk again with the couple or at least make a referral. Some students may say the physician is within his rights to refuse the case since the parents refuse to follow his recommendations.

6. What is the nurse's responsibility to ensure follow-up care?
See answer 3. The nurse could also confront the physician and say she is going to recommend a referral because she is afraid of a lawsuit.

SUGGESTED RESPONSES TO CASE STUDY II

Mr. Thomas is an eighty-nine-year-old resident in a long-term care facility. Mr. Thomas has a long history of diabetes with many complications. At present, he is losing his eyesight and has gangrene in his right foot. Mr. Thomas' family consists of two children, a son and a daughter, who visit for short periods every couple of weeks. Mr. Thomas says they are very busy running the business he started. Mr. Thomas' wife died four years ago and he misses her very much as he tells the nurse frequently. The pastor of Mr. Thomas' church visits at least weekly. The nurse has developed a special rapport with Mr. Thomas and he calls the nurse his "special nurse." Mr. Thomas has told the nurse he is ready to die and "does not want any of that stuff done to keep him alive." He asks the nurse to promise not to let them. When the nurse arrives for work, Mr. Thomas has been scheduled for surgery and is to be transferred. The nurse at report said Dr. Jones and Mr. Thomas' children made the decision and Mr. Thomas is not happy but no one is listening to him.

1. What are the moral/ethical issues?
   (1) The patient has a right to choose his care. The Patient Self-Determination Act provides the patient with the right to refuse treatment even if not having the treatment means he may die. The treatment is against the patient's wishes.
   (2) The physician thinks he must provide appropriate care to the patient and is following his belief value system. The physician thinks the surgery is necessary.
   (3) An ethical/moral issue may be Mr. Thomas is depressed about losing his wife and therefore refusing treatment. If so, is he in a frame of mind to make decisions about his care?
   (4) Another moral/ethical issue is does the health care team have the right to not do all they can to improve Mr. Thomas' health? If they do nothing, are they assisting in his death?
   (5) The nurse has a decision to make regarding whether or not to act as an advocate for the client or ignore the client's wishes and allow the physician and family to make the health decisions for Mr. Thomas.

2. Systematically collect and analyze all data and discuss its relevance to the ethical issues.
   The data and ethical issues are stated in the answer to question 1. The instructor can lead students in listing all data and ethical issues they find in the case study and then relate the data to the ethical issues.

3. Are there emotional issues that are clouding the question?
   Mr. Thomas trusted the nurse enough to confide in her. The nurse has developed a special relationship with Mr. Thomas and has bonded with him.

4. What is the dilemma?
   Does the nurse act as an advocate for the client or allow the physician and family to make the decision? Is Mr. Thomas in a sound frame of mind? Is the physician correct in doing the surgery without considering the client's wishes?

5. List all the choices of action.
   (1) The nurse can notify the physician and family of Mr. Thomas' wishes.
   (2) The nurse could call the pastor and see if Mr. Thomas has related specific instructions for physical care to him.

(3) The nurse can remain silent and let the doctor perform surgery.

6. Analyze the advantages and disadvantages of each choice.
   The instructor can lead the students in discussing advantages and disadvantages of all choices the students list.

7. What should you, Mr. Thomas' special nurse, do, if anything?
   The student will have to answer this individually.

ANSWERS TO THE REVIEW QUESTIONS

1. An ethical right is a right that is:
   d. based on moral principle.
2. Nurses would use the Code for Licensed Practical/Vocational Nurses to:
   c. understand the professional expectations required of them.
3. Values influence the nurse-client relationship because:
   b. every individual has a personal value system that helps determine his/her actions and reactions.
4. By observing a client's body language, a nurse discovers that his client is exceptionally modest about undressing for an examination. The nurse should:
   b. respect the client's need for privacy, even if it seems excessive to him.
5. Values clarification is a useful exercise for the nurse to perform because it:
   a. helps the nurse make ethically sound decisions.
6. An ethical dilemma is:
   c. a problem with two equally bad solutions.

CHAPTER 4
Biomedical Ethics

SUGGESTED RESPONSES TO THE CASE STUDY

Mrs. C. has been admitted to the hospital for treatment of a blood clot in her left leg. The following information was collected upon admission.

Mrs. C. is a seventy-eight-year-old woman who has enjoyed fairly good health most of her life. She is a widow who never had children. There are no living relatives. She does not have an advance directive, nor has she discussed her wishes for health care with any friends, her physician, or clergy. Mrs. C. regularly attended the Methodist church but due to her declining health, has not attended routinely for the last six months.

On day two of her admission, Mrs. C. experiences a cerebral bleed which is exacerbated by the blood thinning medication she is receiving for her blood clot. Mrs. C. slips into a semicomatose state.

1. List subjective data a nurse would assess to verify the client's competency.
   Assess client's state of consciousness, orientation, and awareness.

2. List two persons who could give consent for Mrs. C.
   In an emergency situation, the physician can go ahead with treatment. A judge, through a court order, can give consent for Mrs. C.

3. Write one nursing diagnosis and goal for Mrs. C.
   Communication impaired, verbal, related to cerebral bleed as evidenced by a semicomatose state. Mrs. C. will regain ability to communicate verbally.

4. List two ethical principles that apply in this case.
   Nonmaleficence and beneficence.

5. How can the nurse act as the client advocate for Mrs. C?
   The nurse can act as the client advocate for Mrs. C. by making sure she receives considerate and respectful care.

ANSWERS TO REVIEW QUESTIONS

1. How can nurses protect the privacy of the client?
   a. Monitoring who has access to the chart.
2. Interventions that nurses can use to support efficiency in health care include:
   b. using a preventative approach to care.
3. Sources of organ donors are:
   b. family members.
4. Active euthanasia means a person:
   a. helps a client to die.

CHAPTER 5

Communication

SUGGESTED RESPONSES TO CASE STUDY

Martha, a twenty-five-year-old Mexican-American female, is admitted for severe abdominal pain. Martha clung onto her mother's arm when the nurse asked the mother to leave the room during the admission procedure. The mother asked to stay in the room. The nurse looked to Martha who smiled but said nothing.

1. What subjective and objective data should the nurse gather?
   Subjective data: **Can Martha hear? Ask about the pain, anxiety, fear.**
   Objective data: **Does she speak English? Can she speak? Abdominal tenderness or distention. Date of last bowel movement. Location and type of pain, bowel sounds.**

2. What may be causing Martha to cling to her mother?
   She cannot hear; she cannot speak; she is in so much pain and frightened; she has mental retardation.

3. What can the nurse do to communicate with Martha?
   Ask questions directly to Martha, speaking slowly and distinctly in a normal tone of voice. Give Martha paper and pencil. If no response, ask Martha's mother to assist in the communication.

4. Identify a nursing diagnosis for Martha.
   Fear, related to pain and unfamiliar situation; pain, related to tissue trauma; risk for impaired verbal communication, related to impaired speech ability

ANSWERS TO THE REVIEW QUESTIONS

1. Mr. George is looking out the window with his back to the door. A nurse opens the door and says, "You will not be able to eat or drink after supper because of tests tomorrow." Then the nurse leaves. Did communication take place?
   a. No, there was no feedback.
2. What is the best way to communicate?
   c. It depends on what the message is.
3. Initial client assessment related to communication would include:
   b. visual deficits.
4. When performing a nursing procedure on a client the nurse should:
   b. be aware of her own nonverbal messages.
5. The nurse is aware that most nursing procedures are performed in which spatial comfort zone?
   d. intimate
6. Which of the following is the best way for a nurse to show caring?
   c. assist the client to learn self care.
7. A terminally ill client denies that there is anything wrong and talks constantly about going back to work. The nurse should:
   b. acknowledge the hopes and wishes.
8. The nurse uses therapeutic communication with the client to:
   c. obtain or provide information.
9. The nurse is aware that communication among members of the health care team is necessary because it:
   a. provides for continuity of care.
10. Mrs. Banc tells the nurse that she would rather die than have radiation. To whom should the nurse report this communication?
    c. the physician and charge nurse.

CHAPTER 6
Cultural Aspects of Health and Illness

SUGGESTED RESPONSES TO THE CASE STUDY

Jose Santiago is a fifty-seven-year-old migrant worker who was brought to the evening screening clinic by his crew leader. The crew leader reported that Jose had collapsed in a cucumber field at 4:30 P.M. after ten hours of work and a midday sun temperature of 96°F.
Physical findings included:
BP = 140/86; P = 120; R = 24; T = 102°F
Height = 68˝; Weight = 220 lbs.
Skin: Hot, red, dry
A diagnosis of heat stroke is made. A cool bath reduces the temperature to 100.8°. Mr. Santiago refuses hospitalization and is sent home with a prescription for diazepam (Valium) 10 mg t.i.d., and instructions to monitor temperature and pulse q.i.d., and bed rest for two days. The community health nurse visited Mr. Santiago the next day and found him working in the cucumber field. In talking with him, she learns he visited the local healer during the night and did not get his prescription filled.

1. What are the most likely reasons Mr. Santiago returned to work the day after having a heat stroke?
He had faith in the ability of the faith healer to heal him. He received no sick pay so he could not afford not to work. He perceived it to be the duty of man to work and provide for his family.

2. Discuss the community health nurse's response to Mr. Santiago upon learning he visited the local healer and did not fill his prescription for diazepam.
Possible responses:
(1) She was probably disappointed and frustrated.
(2) She could inquire as to the reason for not getting the prescription filled—financial, beliefs about taking medicine, no transportation, etc.

3. Assess the health beliefs and practices of Mr. Santiago using the Cultural Assessment Guide (refer to Table 6-3, category 6).
Compare beliefs of Mexican-Americans to the Cultural Assessment Guide.

4. Write three individualized nursing diagnoses and goals for Mr. Santiago. Include one culturally related nursing diagnosis.
***Nursing Diagnosis 1:* noncompliance related to cultural beliefs**
***Goal:* Mr. Santiago will discuss his cultural beliefs as they relate to the prescribed medical regimens.**
***Nursing Diagnosis 2:* Risk for fluid volume deficit related to extreme exposure to heat**
***Goal:* Mr. Santiago will demonstrate no symptoms of dehydration.**
***Nursing Diagnosis 3:* Hyperthermic related to sun exposure**
***Goal:* Mr. Santiago's temperature will return to a normal level.**

5. List resources specific to location that could assist Mr. Santiago.
Answers will vary according to location. Possible resources may be migrant health clinic, migrant worker's crew leader and/or boss, local pharmacy for indigent farm worker's organization

6. Describe the teaching that Mr. Santiago will need.
Avoid long periods of exposure to excessive heat. If work demands being in the sun, increase fluid intake and wear a straw hat to shield head from sun. Splash cool water on face when working in the sun. Drink electrolyte balance liquid. Place a cool, wet towel around neck when working in the sun.

7. List at least three successful client outcomes for Mr. Santiago.
(1) Mr. Santiago utilized appropriate medical measures to treat his diagnosis of heat stroke.
(2) Mr. Santiago related signs and symptoms of dehydration and three measures to prevent dehydration from occurring.
(3) Mr. Santiago maintained a lowered body temperature after medical treatment.

ANSWERS TO THE REVIEW QUESTIONS

1. The LP/VN who believes all clients would think about illness the way he/she does is
d. ethnocentric.
2. The LP/VN who believes all immigrants should assume an "American" outlook toward health is demonstrating
a. acculturation.
3. Which of the following is a characteristic of culture?
a. culture is learned.
4. Which of the following is descriptive of Hispanic Americans?
c. illness may be a punishment from God.
5. When an African American says to the nurse, "I need to pray with my pastor in order to get well," the most appropriate response from the nurse is:
c. "May I call your pastor for you and ask him to visit you?"
6. It is important to be aware of cultural aspects of health and disease because:
b. cultural groups respond differently to illness.
7. Which of the following statements is true about the distribution of ethnic groups in the United States?
c. Hispanics are increasing at a greater rate than whites.

CHAPTER 7

Cultural Diversity in the Workplace

SUGGESTED RESPONSES TO THE CASE STUDY

Maria Garcia brings her Catholic, eighteen-year-old sister, Rosa, to the hospital emergency room with a high temperature, chills, vomiting, and complaint of right lower quadrant pain. She brings her three children, ages 3, 2, and 1 year old, with her. Maria understands and speaks broken English, but Rosa is fluent in Spanish only. The nurse directs Maria to the waiting room with her children, then takes Rosa to the examination room. Rosa is examined by a male nurse who promptly complains at the nurses' station about how uncooperative Rosa was with the physical examination. Rosa is admitted for inpatient care with a diagnosis of appendicitis requiring emergency surgery. Maria is left in the waiting room unaware of the difficulty the nursing staff has had communicating with Rosa. Rosa is taken upstairs to her room to await her surgical preparation. Maria is notified that she can go upstairs for a few minutes but must then leave because her children do not meet the age requirement for visitor privileges. Maria finds Rosa weeping and nearly hysterical. The physician walks in and asks Maria why she waited so long to bring Rosa in for treatment. He informs her that Rosa's appendix was close to rupturing and that treatment should have been started three days ago when her symptoms first began. Maria informs him that she had taken Rosa to the curandero, who had given her some herbal tea to drink, but that when it did not help she had brought Rosa to the hospital.

1. Why was communication between Maria, Rosa, and the health care professionals a problem?
    Communication between Maria, Rosa, and the health care professionals was a problem for a number of reasons. First, no effort was made to utilize a translator for Rosa, who is fluent in Spanish only, and for Maria, who understands and speaks broken English. Second, health care professionals made no attempt to include Maria in the room while they were examining and questioning Rosa. Third, the physician's approach to Maria was very blunt and tactless. His accusations of delaying medical treatment were very alienating to Maria.

2. What Mexican-American cultural diversities were not addressed by the health care professionals?
    Several Mexican-American cultural diversities were not addressed by the health care professionals. Several of these include: Rosa was examined by a male nurse and females from the Mexican-American culture generally do not want male nurses or doctors to examine them; family plays a primary role in the health care decisions, but Maria was kept out of the ER and not informed of her sister's admission until she was already admitted to her room. No attempt was made to accommodate for Maria to visit Rosa with her three small children.

3. What needs of Maria and Rosa are being ignored by the health care professionals?
    Rosa has not been given culturally appropriate care: she was examined by a male nurse and physician; she was not afforded informed consent for treatment or admission since no efforts were made to provide an interpreter. She was separated from her family in a foreign environment and had no way to communicate with them. Maria has also not been treated with respect. She was not informed of her sister's examination and results in the ER. She was not given the opportunity for an interpreter to explain to her the situation of Rosa's medical condition and plan for care. The physician's communication style has been inappropriate and disrespectful.

4. What questions do you feel need to be asked by the health care professionals to give them a better understanding of this situation?
    Would you like us to get a Spanish-speaking interpreter for you? If yes, then the interpreter could have asked the following questions: Would you be more comfortable with a female nurse and doctor? Has Rosa ever been admitted to a hospital before? Do Rosa and Maria understand the

diagnosis and plan for treatment? Is there anyone else you would like us to call before you give us permission for treatment? How can we help you make provisions for child care for Maria's children? How does the herbal tea help? Has the *curandero* been helpful in the past? What other treatment plans have you followed at home besides drinking herbal tea?

5. Write three individualized culturally sensitive nursing diagnoses and goals for Rosa.
   Nursing Diagnosis 1: **Verbal communication impaired, related to foreign language barriers.**
   Goal: **Using a Spanish-speaking interpreter, Rosa will communicate understanding of her condition and treatment plan.**
   Nursing Diagnosis 2: **Spiritual distress, potential for, related to separation from religious and cultural ties.**
   Goal: **Rosa will verbalize through the interpreter her feelings of spiritual distress.**
   Nursing Diagnosis 3: **Anxiety related to situational crisis.**
   Goal: **Rosa will verbalize potential and actual sources of anxiety to an interpreter.**

6. Recalling the diagnoses and goals identified in question 5, list pertinent nursing interventions for Rosa.
   (1) **Contact social services for a Spanish-speaking interpreter. Determine the information the family needs. Talk more slowly than usual to Maria. Enlist Maria's help to make flashcards to improve communication with Rosa when an interpreter is unavailable. Using a Spanish-speaking interpreter, explain to Rosa and Maria the treatment plan and clarify their understanding of it.**
   (2) **Listen for cues that Rosa may be having spiritual distress (such as, "Why did God do this to me?" or "What have I done to bring this upon me?"). Remain nonjudgmental. Acknowledge spiritual concerns and encourage the expression of thoughts and feelings. Encourage Rosa to continue her religious practices during hospitalization and do whatever is necessary to help facilitate this (respect rosary beads, crucifix, and Spanish prayer book, look for Spanish mass on television). Ask Rosa if she desires to have a priest visit, and contact the parish if necessary.**
   (3) **Spend time with Rosa to allow verbalization of her fears, discomfort using flashcards, or sign language. Use the universal sign of caring, a smile. Encourage independence. Include Rosa in decisions related to her care whenever possible. Include family in decision making as well. Allow the family to spend as much time with Rosa as possible. Give Rosa, through an interpreter, clear, concise explanations of anything that is about to occur. Plan ahead so that this explanation can be given when the interpreter is at the bedside or use the telephone if necessary.**

7. List resources that the nurses could use to assist Rosa in her recovery.
   AT&T Language line services (800-752-6096) for telephone interpretation; books on communicating with Hispanic clients; hospital-provided Spanish interpreter; priest or nun from Rosa's parish; picture flash cards; Rosa's family members; language conversion dictionary, or printed sheets.

8. List at least three successful client outcomes for Rosa.
   Rosa will establish effective communication with health care provider; Rosa will express satisfaction that her spiritual needs are being met; Rosa will display decreased level of anxiety.

ANSWERS TO REVIEW QUESTIONS

1. Select the trait to avoid when studying about persons of different cultures.
   c. stereotyping
2. A mother is observed breast-feeding her four-year-old son who is a client in the pediatrics wing of the hospital. A nurse is overheard talking in the nursing station about the weird ways the mother has continuing to breast-feed a four-year-old. She comments that the American way is the best. The nurse is guilty of:
   a. ethnocentrism.
3. Which religious group teaches that physical healing exclusively comes through prayers and readings?
   c. Christian Science.
4. Which religious group observes the Sabbath from sunset Friday until sunset Saturday?
   b. Jews

5. A client of this religious denomination would most likely refuse a blood transfusion even if his life was in jeopardy.
    b. Jehovah's Witness
6. The nursing diagnosis that might be used for a client who is hospitalized and has religious practices that are difficult to maintain is:
    c. spiritual distress.
7. It is important for the nurse to know the client's religion in order to:
    b. give holistic care.
8. The kosher practice refers to:
    d. Jewish dietary laws.

CHAPTER 8
Health Maintenance

SUGGESTED ANSWERS FOR THE CASE STUDY

Use the genogram in Figure 8-4. The individual has a high level administrative position at a large university. He must attend many luncheon and dinner meetings. Free time is spent reading novels or watching TV.

1. Identify the possible health problems for the individual.
    Angina, heart disease, stroke, atherosclerosis, diabetes mellitus, hypertension
2. List the lifestyle changes the individual must make to lower his risk of health problems.
    Quit smoking; exercise 30 minutes 3–5 times a week; eat a low-fat, low-cholesterol, high-fiber diet; practice relaxation or meditation.
3. Identify secondary preventive measures the individual should take.
    Have a yearly physical exam including a testicular exam, rectal exam of prostate, EKG, CBC, blood sugar, cholesterol, urine analysis, and stool for blood. Have regular blood pressure checks.
4. Identify the possible health problems for the children.
    Hypertension, heart disease, stroke
5. List ways the children can lower their risk for the health problems identified in statement 4.
    Children 1 and 3—Lose weight; eat a reduced sodium, low-fat, low-cholesterol, high-fiber diet; exercise 30 minutes three to five times a week; do not start smoking.
    Children 2 and 4—maintain appropriate weight for height; eat a reduced sodium, low-fat, low-cholesterol, high-fiber diet; exercise 30 minutes three to five times a week; do not start smoking.
6. Identify the secondary preventive measures the children should be taking.
    Child 1—Physical exam every one to two years, breast exam yearly, baseline mammogram, EKG, Pap smear, CBC, blood sugar, cholesterol, urine analysis, and stool for blood.
    Children 2, 3, and 4—Physical exam every one to three years including testicular exam, EKG, CBC, blood sugar, cholesterol, urine analysis, and stool for blood.

ANSWERS TO THE REVIEW QUESTIONS

1. The person responsible for health maintenance and disease prevention is the:
    c. individual.
2. The *Healthy People 2000* objectives:
    d. address the issue of personal responsibility for health behaviors.

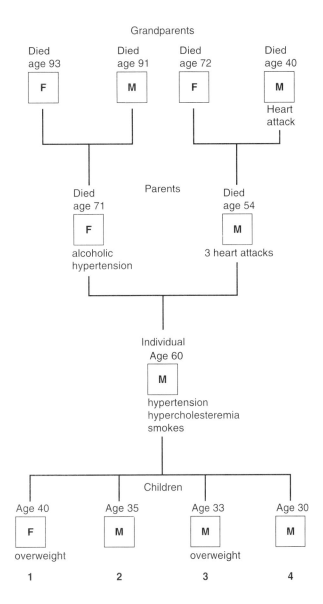

Grandparents

Died age 93 — F
Died age 91 — M
Died age 72 — F
Died age 40 — M
Heart attack

Parents

Died age 71 — F
alcoholic
hypertension

Died age 54 — M
3 heart attacks

Individual
Age 60 — M
hypertension
hypercholesteremia
smokes

Children

Age 40 — F
overweight
1

Age 35 — M
2

Age 33 — M
overweight
3

Age 30 — M
4

FIGURE 8-4 Genogram for case study

3. Primary prevention:
   c. takes place before disease begins.
4. The prevention health care team is composed of the:
   b. individual, physician, and nurses.
5. Health is improved by:
   a. not smoking.
6. How often should an individual have a physical exam?
   d. it depends on the person's age
7. A genogram is used for:
   b. identifying potential health problems.
8. Colds and flu can best be prevented by:
   c. washing hands frequently.
9. Cataracts can be prevented by:
   b. wearing sunglasses and a hat.
10. What is the secondary prevention for stress?
    a. use professional help

CHAPTER 9
Substance Abuse

SUGGESTED RESPONSES TO THE CASE STUDY

Joe, age nineteen, quit school three years ago. He has a part-time job at a fast food place but has been tardy or absent quite often lately. Sometimes he is easy to get along with, and sometimes he is aggressive and difficult. His mother, with whom he lives, says he is a good boy and does not give her any trouble. Joe was brought to the emergency room by a friend after he passed out. His temperature is 99°F, respirations 10, and pupils are pinpoint. There are track marks on both arms.

1. List signs and symptoms, other than Joe's, that a client may experience as a heroin addict.
   Other signs and symptoms may include euphoria, constipation, and orthostatic hypotension.

2. List diagnostic tests that may be ordered.
   A drug screening test may be ordered.

3. List subjective and objective data the nurse should obtain.
   Subjective data: behavioral changes, problems at work or home, legal problems (DWI), how often drugs are used, how much is used.
   Objective data: appearance, personal care (cleanliness, bad breath, dental caries, nutritional status), condition of nasal mucosa, depressed respirations, track marks on arms, tremors, slurred speech, lack of coordination, jaundice, frequent episodes of sexually transmitted diseases, appearance older than stated age.

4. Write three individualized nursing diagnoses and goals for Joe.
   ***Nursing Diagnosis 1:* Injury, high risk for, related to altered cerebral function.**
   ***Goal:* Joe will not be injured because of passing out from drugs.**
   ***Nursing Diagnosis 2:* Infection, high risk for, related to site for invasion of organism.**
   ***Goal:* Joe will not get an infection in the track marks on his arm.**
   ***Nursing Diagnosis 3:* Family coping, compromised, ineffective related to mother's denial of problem.**
   ***Goal:* Joe will communicate with his mother, sharing his concerns and activities.**

5. List resources within the medical center and local area that could assist Joe.
   Resources may include individual or group counseling, drug treatment center, Narcotics Anonymous.

6. Describe the use of methadone in heroin addiction.
   Methadone is used to assist users of heroin cease using heroin. Methadone keeps the withdrawal symptoms under control. Random and routine urine drug screening is done to assure compliance.

7. List teaching that Joe will need as part of his rehabilitation.
   Joe will need to be taught adaptive coping methods to handle life's stressors.

ANSWERS TO REVIEW QUESTIONS

1. Schedule II substances:
   b. have high abuse and dependence potential.

2. Substance use and abuse are:
   a. influenced by advertising.

3. Prevention of substance abuse must be focused on:
   b. children.

4. Drug screening tests:
   c. indicate exposure to a substance.
5. The substance most often chosen for abuse or dependence is:
   c. alcohol.
6. Alcoholics Anonymous is:
   d. a self-help group providing a holistic approach to abstinence.
7. Urinary acidifiers are used in the treatment of:
   b. amphetamines and PCP.
8. The use of inhalants:
   a. can be fatal.

CHAPTER 10

Nursing Assessment

SUGGESTED RESPONSES TO THE CASE STUDY

Tom Turner, age forty, was admitted to the hospital with pneumonia. He had never been hospitalized before. His wife and three children are at home. Because his wife has just given birth to their third child, Tom's wife cannot drive the other two children to school. Tom provides the sole income for the family, and he only has three more sick days to use at work before he will be off without pay.

Tom's vital signs are BP 120/72, P 100, R 34, T 106°F. His breath sounds show sonorous wheezes throughout, cleared by coughing. His cough is frequent and productive of foamy, cloudy, yellow secretions. His AP is 102 and regular, but distant heart tones were noted. The abdomen is firm and distended with hypoactive bowel sounds noted in all four quadrants. He moves all extremities slowly but per self and with purpose.

Tom is oriented to person, place, and time. His pupils are PERRLA. Hand grips are strong and equal bilaterally, as are foot pushes. He speaks only when spoken to, and his eye contact with staff is minimal. Whenever his wife visits, his voice raises and his heart rate increases about 2-5 beats. At one point, Tom stated, "How much more of this can we take?" Tom's wife mentions that their church would love to help, but Tom refuses to take charity. Tom states, "Any income for this family has to come from me."

Other added information acquired during the assessment included the fact that Tom has a history of drinking 1 to 2 beers daily, and has not performed testicular self-exams. He eats and drinks what he likes, and he states he really "hates seafood." Usually he bathes daily in the early morning and helps to bathe two of their children each evening. His job is 9–5:30 P.M., five days per week, and also some Saturday mornings. Tom pays all of the household bills, and is the sole decision maker of the family.

1. List the functional assessment data collected from Mr. Turner that identify psychosocial concerns.
   Eye contact is minimal.
   Voice raises and heart rate increases 2–5 beats when wife is present.
2. List the data supporting Mr. Turner's diagnosis of pneumonia.
   Sonorous wheezes.
   Cough frequent and productive of foamy, cloudy, yellow secretions.
   Respirations 34
   Temperature 100.6

3. What are two possible reasons for identifying the added information about Mr. Turner in the last paragraph?
    May be signs of future physical health problems. May be signs of future mental health problems.

4. Write two or three nursing diagnoses that are supported by the health history and physical assessments documented about Mr. Turner.
    Breathing pattern, ineffective, related to pneumonia as evidenced by R 34, sonorous wheezes, and productive cough.
    Health maintenance, altered, related to lack of preventive health care as evidenced by no testicular self-exams, daily beer, and eating and drinking what he likes.

5. Write goals and nursing interventions for each nursing diagnosis.
    Mr. Turner will have normal rate of respiration, breath sounds clear and no cough.
    Administer medications as ordered.
    Encourage expectoration of coughing products.
    Encourage some activity between periods of rest.
    Mr. Turner will perform monthly testicular self-exam.
    Teach Mr. Turner how to perform testicular self-exam.
    Provide literature on testicular self-exam.

6. The priority actions to be taken for Mr. Turner while he is in the hospital focus specifically on which functional patterns?
    Health perception/Health management
    Coping/Stress tolerance

7. List at least two ways the nurse could evaluate Mr. Turner's physical recovery from pneumonia.
    Breath sounds clear
    No cough

ANSWERS TO THE REVIEW QUESTIONS

1. Jim's apical pulse is 102. He states to the nurse that he can feel his heart pounding. Which of the following charting terms would accurately describe Jim's statement of concern regarding his heart rate?
    c. palpitation

2. Mrs. Jones is fifty-four years old. While performing your assessment overview, Mrs. Jones states, "I just get so lightheaded when I first get up in the morning." Mrs. Jones most likely has:
    d. orthostatic hypotension.

3. According to Gordon's Eleven Functional Health Patterns, which pattern focuses on: the health and wellness of the person, performance of self-exams, lifestyle, and habits that could influence a person's state of wellness?
    b. health perception-health management

4. During the physical head-to-toe assessment of the client, the nurse checks his pulse and blood pressure. Which of the four assessment techniques did the nurse utilize?
    c. auscultation and palpation

5. The client and the nurse were discussing the following data. In which of the eleven functional health patterns would you place the majority of this data?
    • abdomen firm, distended, hypoactive bowel sounds
    • eats and drinks what he likes
    • states he really hates seafood
    • Temperature 100.6°F
    • bathes daily in the early A.M.
    d. nutritional-metabolic

6. The nurse is collecting health history and physical assessment data about a newly admitted twelve-year-old girl experiencing difficulty breathing. Of the data listed below, which would be of lowest priority?
    d. weight and height

7. Upon admission to your unit, the client verbalizes an increased pain in her left leg. What would be the pertinent assessment information to collect about this client?
    c. assess both of the client's legs

8. Which of the pulses should be assessed when trying to identify good circulation to the lower extremities?
    a. dorsalis pedis

9. How often a nurse assesses a client's vital signs depends upon:
   d. client's condition.
10. The nurse checks the radial pulse for 30 seconds and multiplies by 2. She notices an irregularity in the beat. What is the next action the nurse should take?
    b. Listen to the apical pulse for 60 seconds.

CHAPTER 11

Anesthesia

SUGGESTED RESPONSES TO THE CASE STUDY

Mrs. Jones is in the recovery room following outpatient surgery. She had a general anesthetic and is now awake, breathing deeply, and talking to the staff. She has received meperidine (Demerol) intravenously and is quite comfortable. Before being discharged home from the day surgery center Mrs. Jones rests in an easy chair in the transitional recovery area. The nurse taking care of her notices that she asks questions about things that have already been discussed and has even asked one question three times.

1. After making these observations what nursing diagnoses and goals might the nurse identify for Mrs. Jones?

2. List the nursing interventions to be performed in caring for Mrs. Jones.

3. Identify how teaching should be done.
   (1) A preexisting neurological problem could account for Mrs. Jones's difficulty remembering things after her anesthetic. Presuming that Mrs. Jones had a normal memory prior to her anesthetic, the nurse should remember that anesthetic and sedative drugs cause temporary amnesia and that her lack of memory may persist for minutes to hours after the anesthetic even if she appears to be completely recovered in other ways.
   Nursing Diagnosis 1: **Injury, high risk for, related to amnesiac effect of anesthesia and sedative drugs.**
   Goal: **Mrs. Jones will not be injured.**
   (2) Nursing interventions for nursing diagnosis 1: Watch Mrs. Jones closely. She may forget being instructed not to get out of the chair by herself and try to get up to go to the bathroom or get a drink of water. The effects of either the surgical procedure or the anesthetic may result in a fall and an injury to Mrs. Jones.
   (1) *Nursing Diagnosis 2:* **Thought processes, altered, related to anesthesia as evidenced by asking questions about things already discussed.**
   Goal: **Mrs. Jones will express understanding of instructions.**
   (2, 3) Nursing interventions for nursing diagnosis 2: Go over Mrs. Jones's discharge instructions in the presence of the individual responsible for taking her home and caring for her that day. Although they are written down, clients and caregivers often have questions about their instructions. Mrs. Jones may ask questions while the instructions are being explained yet be unable to remember the nurses' answers later in the day.

ANSWERS TO REVIEW QUESTIONS

1. Who is qualified to explain anesthesia and its risks and benefits in a manner sufficient to secure an informed consent from a client or their legal guardian?
   b. an anesthetist or surgeon

2. Why are clients at risk for aspiration of gastric contents into the lungs when they have a general anesthetic?
   b. General anesthesia eliminates protective airway reflexes.
3. What is the most important result of oversedation?
   d. inability to breathe adequately
4. What is the most convincing sign that a client has a post dural puncture headache following a spinal or epidural regional anesthetic?
   c. It gets worse when the client sits up or stands.
5. In addition to keeping the client unconscious, preventing the sensation of pain, and relaxing muscles to hold the client still and allow for surgical exposure, what does an anesthetist do to ensure a safe anesthetic?
   a. control vital functions like breathing and heart rate
6. How long after a general anesthetic might it be before a client can think as clearly as before the client had an anesthetic?
   d. several days
7. What effect might a spinal or epidural anesthetic still have after normal sensation and motor function have returned?
   b. decrease in blood pressure when the client stands up (orthostatic hypotension)

CHAPTER 12

Pain Management

SUGGESTED RESPONSES TO THE CASE STUDY

Johnny Prince, a twenty-seven-year-old male, is admitted to the medical unit diagnosed with hemophilia and septic arthritis in his left ankle. He has a history of epilepsy, arthritis, artificial knee joints (bilateral), and two hip surgeries. Medications taken at home include: factor VIII, phenobarbital 100 mg hs, and Naprosyn 5 mg t.i.d. His chief complaint is swelling and severe pain in his left ankle.

CURRENT RX: *Colace, MOM, ceftriaxon sodium (Rocephin) IV piggy-back, phenobarbital 100 mg q hs, $FeSO_4$, multivitamins, vitamin C, oxacillin (Bactocill), factor VIII 20,000 IVP q 12 hrs, hydromorphone HCl (Dilaudid) 8 mg po q 8 hrs (hold SBP < 90, resp. < 12), MS 4 mg IVP q 4 hrs prn, flurazepam HCl (Dalmane) 30 mg po q hs prn.*

1. What will you include in assessing Mr. Prince's pain?
   Subjective data: Location of pain, onset and duration, quality (using his own words), intensity (on a scale of 0–10), aggravating and relieving factors, how pain is affecting his activities of daily living. Objective data: changes in vital signs, swelling and temperature of skin, and ROM in left ankle. Note any pain behaviors (e.g., moaning, guarding).

2. What factors in his history will influence his pain perception?
   Johnny has lived with joint pain most of his life, due to hemophilia. He has had arthritis, especially in knees and hips (shown by his surgeries). Since he has lived with chronic pain, he may not show signs of acute pain (e.g., changes in vital signs).

   Your pain assessment gives you the following information:
   * *Location—through center of ankle*
   * *Intensity—pain at time of assessment is 5 (medicated thirty minutes prior to interview) on scale of 0–10, at its worse = 25, at its best = 3.*

- *Quality—describes pain as throbbing at times, a jabbing pain. It hurts worse between 9 and 10 A.M. and 9 and 12 at night. Mainly worse when medicine wears off.*
- *Effects of pain—only gets two or three hrs of sleep, often dreaming about it. Pain makes him avoid activity, gets grumpy and snappy. Concentration turns totally to pain.*
- *Behaviors—he yells at times, but doesn't like to. He'd prefer to "sweat it out." Also grimaces, grips hands and tries repositioning.*

3. Why did the physician order the analgesics on that schedule?

   Johnny has constant pain; therefore, the physician ordered Dilaudid to be administered on a scheduled basis (ATC) to prevent pain and maintain drug level. The morphine is for breakthrough pain.

4. Mr. Prince requests a dose of morphine. The narcotic drawer has the following available in prefilled syringe cartridges: 2 mg per cc, and 8 mg per cc. Which cartridge(s) should the nurse select?

   Select the 8 mg per cc, and waste one-half cc.

5. Why is the morphine ordered IVP, not IM?

   With Mr. Prince's diagnosis of hemophilia, he should not receive IM injections. Also, IVP provides a more rapid onset of relief for severe pain.

6. Why did the physician order colace and MOM?

   The physician was concerned about the constipation that occurs with opioid use. The client's immobility due to a painful ankle would further exacerbate this problem.

7. What are some noninvasive relief measures that might be tried with Mr. Prince?

   Ice packs applied to the ankle may give relief from the swelling and pain. Relaxation and imagery could provide relief for current pain problem, plus teach coping skills that could be used in the future. Massage would not be appropriate due to his hemophilia, which may increase bleeding. Distraction may provide relief for procedural pain, but would not provide long-term relief.

8. What can the nurse do, using medications from current orders, to promote better sleeping patterns for Mr. Prince?

   Administer morphine and Dalmane together at hour of sleep, give second morphine dose four hours later, even if Mr. Prince is still sleeping. This may prevent the pain from waking him, rather than keeping him awake. Also, use noninvasive techniques discussed above prior to hour of sleep, especially relaxation and guided imagery. This may help promote rest and sleep.

9. Write three individualized nursing diagnoses and goals for Mr. Prince.

   Nursing Diagnosis 1: **Pain, acute, related to inflammatory process of bleeding within ankle joint.**
   Goal: **Mr. Prince will verbalize pain relief as evidenced by a pain rating less than 4 on a scale of 0–10 within 12 hours.**
   Nursing Diagnosis 2: **Knowledge deficit (pain medications) related to misconceptions regarding use of analgesics.**
   Goal: **Mr. Prince will state the importance of preventing pain before the intensity gets too severe within 12 hours.**
   Nursing Diagnosis 3: **Anxiety (moderate) related to unrelieved pain and recurrence of complications.**
   Goal: **Mr. Prince will verbalize a reduction in his anxiety level within 24 hours.**

10. What teaching will Mr. Prince need before discharge?

    Mr. Prince will need to be taught the importance of taking his NSAIDS on a scheduled basis. The importance of relieving pain before it gets severe, rather than "sweating it out," should be reinforced. Relaxation techniques and use of cold packs should be reviewed. Signs and symptoms of further internal bleeding should be reviewed, including instructions on contacting his physician.

ANSWERS TO REVIEW QUESTIONS

1. According to McCaffery, pain may be defined as:

   c. whatever the patient says it is, whenever and wherever the patient says it does.

2. Which of the following is a useful tool for assessing the intensity of pain that is easy to use?

   c. numeric pain scale.

3. Mr. Levy, forty-five, has experienced chronic low back pain since a fall eight years ago. He describes his pain as "a gnawing, constant dull pain" that makes him feel tired. The nurse caring for him recognizes that one of the differences between acute and chronic pain characteristics is:
    b. chronic pain is often described as dull and is difficult to localize.

4. Mrs. Nancy Johnson, eighty-four years old, is recuperating from a total hip replacement. Morphine, 8 mg IV q 4 hours prn, is prescribed for Mrs. Johnson. Her respiratory rate is 18, her pulse rate is 96 beats per minute, and her blood pressure is elevated slightly above her normal level. She is complaining of severe pain, 8 on a scale of 0–10. The most appropriate initial nursing intervention is:
    c. administer the medication as ordered.

5. Ms. Redgrave, fifty-five years old, is hospitalized with an exacerbation of rheumatoid arthritis. She has a favorite television show she watches every afternoon. She reports feeling comfortable during this show and seldom requests pain medication when she is watching it. The nurse's assessment of this phenomenon is that:
    c. inactivity is the best approach to Ms. Redgrave's pain.

6. At what anatomical site does perception of the pain occur?
    d. cortex.

7. One of the general principles of pain management is:
    a. anticipated or mild pain is easier to relieve than severe pain.

CHAPTER 13

Perioperative Nursing

SUGGESTED RESPONSES TO THE CASE STUDY

Mr. Glen Stone, a seventy-four-year-old retired schoolteacher who is married and the father of four and grandfather of sixteen, weighs 275 lbs, has undergone a right hemicolectomy in which the right side of his colon has been removed because of cancer. He has a history of smoking, but has no other health problems. The surgery was uncomplicated and he is in the PACU. He has a midline incision with a Penrose drain and a stab wound with a Jackson Pratt drain adjacent to the incision. He has a nasogastric tube attached to low intermittent suction. He is alert and oriented and moves all four extremities. His blood pressure is normal for him in comparison to preoperative levels. He is breathing regularly and easily at a rate of 16 breaths per minute, has pink mucous membranes, but his oxygen saturation is 86 percent with additional oxygen given via mask.

1. What will you include in assessing risk factors for developing postoperative complications for Mr. Stone?
    Risk factors of Mr. Stone include being elderly, obese, and a smoker.

2. What is his Aldrete Score at this point?
    Mr. Stone's present Aldrete Score is 9.

3. What nursing measures can you institute to promote oxygenation?
    To increase Mr. Stone's level of oxygenation the nurse can: encourage coughing and deep breathing, elevate the head of the bed, and medicate him for pain if needed.

4. What type of drainage is expected from his incision and drains for the first one to two days?
    His incision and drains should drain serosanguinous drainage in decreasing amounts.

5. What nursing observations can be made and reported to indicate to the surgeon that the nasogastric tube can be removed?
    Three observations may indicate that Mr. Stone's nasogastric tube can be removed:

(1) presence of bowel sounds
(2) passing of flatus
(3) decreased quantity of drainage from nasogastric tube

6. What nursing measures can be implemented to prevent deep vein thrombosis, thrombophlebitis, or pulmonary emboli?

Three nursing measures can be implemented to prevent Mr. Stone from developing deep vein thrombosis, thrombophlebitis, and pulmonary embolus:

(1) Ensure continuous and correct use of antiembolism stockings and/or sequential compression device if ordered

(2) Encourage leg exercises

(3) Assist with early ambulation with increasing activity

7. Write three individualized nursing diagnoses and goals for Mr. Stone.

Possible nursing diagnoses for Mr. Stone are:

(1) Gas exchange, impaired, related to smoking, effects of anesthesia, and/or pain as evidenced by oxygen saturation of 86 percent.

(2) Skin integrity, impaired, related to surgery as evidenced by abdominal incision, IV insertion, and drain placement.

(3) Infection, high risk for, related to the invasive procedure, potential fecal contamination, age, obesity, Foley catheter placement, surgical drain placement, and smoking.

(4) Fluid volume deficit, high risk for, related to blood loss and NPO status.

(5) Fluid volume excess, high risk for, related to fluids received during surgery.

(6) Peripheral neurovascular dysfunction, high risk for, related to abdominal surgery, age, obesity, and immobility.

(7) Injury, high risk for, related to anesthesia, weakness, and pain.

(8) Altered nutrition, high risk for, less than body requirements, related to increased protein/vitamin requirements for wound healing and decreased intake secondary to pain, nausea, vomiting, and diet restrictions.

(9) Anxiety, high risk for, related to postoperative diagnosis, possible changes in lifestyle, and alteration in self-concept.

(10) Pain, related to surgical incision and surgical positioning.

8. What information will Mr. Stone need prior to discharge?

Mr. Stone will need information regarding his home medications, diet, activity restrictions, follow-up appointments, wound care, and any other special instructions.

ANSWERS TO THE REVIEW QUESTIONS

1. The nurse, while doing client teaching, implements which one of the following?
   a. Assesses barriers to learning.
2. Client education is:
   d. directed toward the client's family when the client is unable to learn.
3. The role of the nurse in obtaining consent includes which of the following?
   b. Acting as a witness to the signature of the client.
4. The use of drains will:
   d. eliminate fluid accumulation.
5. Upon admission to the PACU, the nurse first:
   b. assesses the airway.
6. The nurse is making a preoperative assessment on a client. Which of these assessments is the most important to know for a client who is having general anesthesia?
   d. a smoker
7. Which of the following persons is responsible and accountable for all activities during a surgical procedure?
   c. circulating nurse
8. The surgical skin preparation will:
   b. cleanse and inhibit bacterial growth.

...ursing intervention that reduces almost all surgical risks is:
...ging activity and early ambulation.
...k increases in the elderly due to:
...ologic aging changes.

CHAPTER 14

Fluid, Electrolyte, and Acid-Base Balances

SUGGESTED RESPONSES TO THE CASE STUDY

Mr. G. R. Calahan is a sixty-seven-year-old retired Army captain who lives with his wife in an apartment over their son's hardware store in a small Midwestern town. Due to behavioral changes throughout the course of the day, his family brought him to the emergency room of the local hospital.

Other than surgeries for an inguinal hernia and hemorrhoids, he has been in good health. Four months ago, during his annual visit to the doctor, his blood pressure was elevated. The diuretic pill prescribed has kept his blood pressure within normal limits. He eats a well-balanced diet, does not smoke, but does like a beer when he is hot. He and his dog go for a two-mile jog each day.

Despite the high humidity and temperature in the nineties, he and his dog went for their usual morning exercise. He had a bowl of oatmeal, a grapefruit, two cups of coffee, and his medication before jogging. When he returned home, he complained of being weak and tired. He apologized for not getting the air conditioner fixed the day before but promised to do it right after his nap. He told his wife he did not feel like eating lunch. He drank a beer to quench his thirst before laying down. Twice he got up to urinate. The second time he almost fell because he was so dizzy. When his son came to visit during the evening meal, he noticed his father was becoming confused and decided to take him to the emergency room.

Serum blood tests revealed elevated hematocrit, electrolytes, and BUN. Although he had been urinating large quantities earlier in the day, he could only produce 30 cc of very concentrated urine in the ER. Specific gravity was 1.025. Mr. Calahan was diagnosed with dehydration.

1. Identify factors that contributed to Mr. Calahan's fluid volume deficit.
   Factors include: age (sixty-seven years old); lack of fluid intake before vigorous exercise; foods/beverages which promote diuresis, i.e., grapefruit, coffee, beer; taking his diuretic pill; and high humidity and atmospheric temperature.

2. What changes in vital signs should the nurse expect to find in a client with a fluid volume deficit?
   Elevated temperature. Low blood pressure, pulse, and respirations.

3. Why are elderly clients especially prone to fluid imbalances?
   Less than 50 percent of their body weight is water; therefore, changes cause problems earlier in the elderly than they would in a younger adult. Renal functioning deteriorates with aging, therefore the body is less able to compensate for imbalances.

4. Discuss why Mr. Calahan's hematocrit is elevated.
   Due to reduction in intravascular fluid.

5. Identify two nursing diagnoses and goals for Mr. Calahan.
    Nursing Diagnosis 1: **Fluid volume deficit, related to excess fluid loss as evidenced by eating grapefruit and drinking coffee and beer.**
    Mr. Calahan will:
    (1) Increase fluid intake to at least 2,000 mL/day.
    (2) Demonstrate a balance between intake and output.
    (3) Not demonstrate any signs or symptoms of a fluid volume deficit.
    Nursing Diagnosis 2: **Knowledge deficit about food and fluid intake related to hot weather, as evidenced by dehydration.**
    Mr. Calahan will drink other fluids (water) when it is very hot.
    Mr. Calahan will have other fruit (melon, grapes) and one cup of coffee when it is very hot.

6. Relate three nursing interventions for a client with a fluid volume deficit.
    Nursing interventions include: careful monitoring of I&O, encourage fluid intake by providing water and liquids within his reach, weigh daily, teach family members causes of fluid deficit and methods to prevent it from occurring.

    An IV of D5NS at 125 cc/hr was started in the ER and he was admitted to a medical unit for future evaluation. When he arrived on the unit, one hour-and-a-half after entering the hospital, the IV site showed no signs of infiltration and 100 cc remained in the bag.

7. Identify a priority nursing diagnosis for Mr. Calahan based upon this information.
    fluid volume excess

8. Identify three nursing interventions the nurse should implement.
    (1) Limit sodium intake
    (2) Monitor I&O
    (3) Weigh daily

9. Relate criteria to use to evaluate the effectiveness of nursing care.
    Intake and output will be equal.
    Daily weight will stay the same.
    Skin turgor will be normal.

10. Identify client teaching to aid in preventing fluid volume deficit during periods of high atmospheric temperature and humidity.
    Limit exposure to heat and humidity; drink at least 2000 mL of fluid a day, avoid foods and beverages that have a diuretic effect, avoid or limit activity during these periods.

ANSWERS TO THE REVIEW QUESTIONS

1. The largest percentage of fluid in the body is located:
    d. within the cells.
2. Diffusion is the movement of:
    b. a solute from an area of high concentration to an area of low concentration.
3. Which of the following foods is high in potassium?
    c. bananas.
4. Clients with hypocalcemia should be encouraged to eat more
    a. broccoli.
5. A pH of 7.41 indicates:
    d. normal pH.
6. Respiratory acidosis develops as a result of:
    a. chronic obstructive pulmonary disease.
7. Diabetics who forget to take their insulin are prone to develop:
    c. metabolic acidosis.

CHAPTER 15
Oncology Nursing

SUGGESTED RESPONSES TO THE CASE STUDY

Mr. John Dalton is a seventy-year-old male with a history of cancer of the prostate, which was treated with palliative hormones and radiation. His admitting diagnosis is adeno-carcinoma of the prostate with widespread bone metastasis. Mr. Dalton is married and has one grown daughter who often helps with his care. His chief complaint is severe back pain. The physician has ordered intrathecal morphine sulfate and aspirin 10 gr. for pain relief.

1. List symptoms typically seen in clients diagnosed with prostate cancer.
   Early symptoms include weak urinary stream, urinary frequency, dysuria and difficulty starting and stopping urination. Some pain may be noted in the lower back, pelvis, or upper thighs. Warning signs include difficulty urinating, painful and frequent urination, and blood in the urine.

2. Identify the population most at risk for developing prostate cancer.
   African-American men.

3. List three possible risk factors for prostate cancer.
   Age, familial association, and studies suggest dietary fat may be a factor.

4. List two types of hormones used in the management of prostate cancer.
   Estrogens, gonadotropin-releasing hormone analogs.

5. Discuss why the physician's orders include aspirin along with morphine sulfate. How do non-narcotic analgesics differ from narcotics?
   Anti-inflammatory drugs inhibit the synthesis of prostaglandins. Prostaglandins are fatty acids found all over the body. The release of prostaglandins in tissue causes pain, edema, and inflammation. By inhibiting the synthesis of prostaglandins, anti-inflammatory drugs decrease inflammation and pain. All cancer clients with bone metastasis should be on aspirin or another non-steroidal anti-inflammatory drug because bone metastasis is inflammatory. Narcotics work on the central nervous system. Non-narcotics work on the periphery.

6. Discuss why benzodiazepines should not be used for pain relief.
   Very few benzodiazepines have analgesic effects and they limit the amount of opioid that can be safely given because of their sedative and respiratory depressant effects.

7. List the subjective and objective data the nurse would want to obtain.
   Subjective data: location and severity of pain, what makes pain worse, dysuria, response to pain medication
   Objective data: color and odor of urine, ability to care for himself, vital signs, I&O, mood swings

8. When you walk into Mr. Dalton's room he greets you with a smile and continues talking and joking with his daughter. While assessing him, you note that his vital signs are normal. You ask him to rate his pain on a scale of 0–10. He pauses to think about it, then rates the pain at 8. In the chart you must record your nursing assessment by circling the appropriate number on the scale. Which number do you think you should circle?
   You should circle 8—the number reported to you. The AHCPR cancer pain guidelines state "the mainstay of pain assessment is the client self-report."

9. Write three individualized nursing diagnoses and goals for Mr. Dalton.
   ***Nursing Diagnosis 1:* Pain, acute, related to tissue trauma.**
   ***Goal:* Mr. Dalton will report pain at <4 within one hour of medication.**
   ***Nursing Diagnosis 2:* Injury, high risk for, related to widespread bone metastases.**
   ***Goal:* Mr. Dalton will not be injured by falling because of receiving medication for bone pain.**

Nursing Diagnosis 3: **Urinary elimination, altered patterns of, high risk for, related to prostate cancer and radiation.**
Goal: **Mr. Dalton will maintain normal pattern of urinary elimination.**

10. Discuss which onocologic emergency Mr. Dalton is most likely to develop.
Spinal cord compression.

ANSWERS TO THE REVIEW QUESTIONS

1. The nurse carefully monitors the client's IV chemotherapy. Which is an early indicator that the extravasation may occur?
d. Burning occurs at the site.

2. A breast cancer client states that the doctor says he is going to prescribe hormone therapy. Which of the following hormones would probably be ordered?
d. testosterone

3. A cancer client develops a low white cell count. She is placed on neutropenic precautions. Which of the following menu selections would be the best choice?
a. meat loaf, mashed potatoes, green beans and fruit gelatin.

4. As stomatitis develops, which would be the best nursing intervention to encourage?
c. Brush teeth after eating and at bedtime.

5. Which nursing action should be encouraged when clients receive radiation?
c. Tell the client not to apply deodorants or lotions while she is receiving radiation.

6. Due to excessive vomiting, the oral route of administration is not possible. Which of the following routes should the nurse consider first?
b. rectal

CHAPTER 16

Caring for the Older Adult

SUGGESTED RESPONSES TO THE CASE STUDY

Mr. Jack Baroni, a seventy-two-year-old male, was admitted to the skilled care facility for rehabilitation following an open reduction, internal fixation of the right hip. Mr. Baroni had fallen while going up the stairs of his home suffering an intertrochanteric, comminuted fracture of the right femur. He has no recollection of what caused him to fall. He is married and until his surgery was working part time as a school-crossing guard. While in the hospital Mr. Baroni exhibited mental status changes including disorientation and confusion. His wife reports that he never had this problem previous to the surgery. He is continent of bowel and bladder. Mr. Baroni was in relatively good health until the fall. He and his wife agree that he should return home after rehabilitation is complete.

1. Identify specific admission assessments that would be required for Mr. Baroni because of his age and condition.
Assessments include risk for pressure ulcers, safety assessment, mini-mental status exam.

2. Identify complications for which Mr. Baroni is at risk.
Complications include thrombophlebitis, pneumonia, pressure ulcers, injury related to falling, and incisional infection.

3. List interventions to prevent each complication.

    Encourage coughing and deep breathing or use incentive spirometer (pneumonia).

    Maintain mobility within the limits of physician's orders (thrombophlebitis).

    Implement a pressure ulcer prevention protocol (pressure ulcers).

    Implement a safety program to prevent falls (injury related to falling).

    Monitor operative site/keep clean/maintain nutrition and hydration to optimize healing conditions (incisional infection).

4. Describe possible reasons causing Mr. Baroni to fall.

    Items on the steps

    Missed the next step

    Blacked out

5. Describe methods for assessing Mr. Baroni's mental status.

    Give a mini-mental status exam shortly after admission. If disorientation continues thereafter, assess orientation by asking him what his plans are for the day.

6. Describe possible reasons for his altered mental status.

    Altered mental status is not uncommon in elderly people after open reduction/internal fixation. It may result from the sudden change in environment (falling, immediate transfer to emergency room, surgery), medications, and anesthesia.

7. Write three individualized nursing diagnoses and goals for Mr. Baroni.

    Thought processes, altered, related to fracture and surgery as evidenced by confusion and disorientation.

    Mr. Baroni will be oriented and not confused.

    Infection, high risk for, related to comminuted fracture, surgery, and age.

    Mr. Baroni will not have an infection in his incision.

    Activity intolerance, high risk for, related to surgery, age, and confusion.

    Mr. Baroni will be able to ambulate in room.

8. List nursing actions related to altered mental status.

    Assess orientation from time to time.

    Avoid restraints by using alternative safety measures.

    Use reality orientation in appropriate ways; calling him by name, explaining what is happening, telling him where he is and why, telling him the date.

    Do not argue with the client or try to "reason" or "use logic" with him if he becomes agitated.

9. List four successful outcomes for Mr. Baroni.

    Mr. Baroni will be able to walk.

    Mr. Baroni will not have any pressure ulcers.

    Mr. Baroni will be oriented and have no confusion.

    Mr. Baroni will have normal breath sounds.

    Mr. Baroni will have no infection.

10. Develop a teaching plan for Mr. Baroni.

    Put clock and large calendar in room.

    When caring for Mr. Baroni, identify the day, date, and time.

    Teach to hold on to stair railing when going up or down stairs.

    Encourage turning in bed to prevent pressure ulcers, pneumonia, and thrombophlebitis.

    Encourage intake of milk and milk products.

    Teach to call for help when able to get out of bed.

11. List the community resources Mr. Baroni may need after discharge.

    Home health nurse once a week to monitor condition, assess general condition and surgical site.

    Physical therapist or physical therapy assistant to continue mobility programs.

    Home health aide 3–4 times a week to provide personal care.

ANSWERS TO REVIEW QUESTIONS

1. Which of the following is a true statement?
   d. Incontinence is not an expected or normal aging change.
2. The programmed aging theory states that:
   b. a genetic clock determines the speed with which people age.
3. The elderly can avoid respiratory tract infections by:
   a. receiving influenza vaccine each year.
4. Research indicates that:
   b. high intensity resistance training can improve muscle strength in the elderly.
5. Aging changes in the skin include:
   d. increased vascular fragility.

CHAPTER 17

Rehabilitation, Home Health, and Long-term Care

SUGGESTED RESPONSES TO THE CASE STUDY

Mrs. Emma James, seventy-two years old, was admitted to Community Hospital for a left below knee amputation. Mrs. James has been an insulin dependent diabetic for thirty-five years. The amputation follows a long and unsuccessful period of treatment for venous stasis ulcers. Mrs. James was transferred from the hospital to a rehabilitation hospital on her fourth postoperative day. After two weeks at the rehabilitation hospital she was transferred to a skilled care facility near her home for additional rehabilitation and regulation of the diabetes. She is now ready to be discharged to her home. Mrs. James has a prosthesis and is able to ambulate with a walker. She can perform her ADL with minimal assistance. She was on a sliding scale and blood glucose monitoring four times a day while in the long-term care facility. Her physician has now placed her on insulin twice a day with daily blood glucose checks. Her vision is somewhat impaired due to the diabetes. Mrs. James lives alone in a one-story home in a safe residential area. The discharge planner at the skilled care facility has arranged continuing care for Mrs. James through a local home health agency.

1. Identify the assessment factors that are most important in planning Mrs. James' care.
   Assessment for risk factors: trauma/injury, pressure ulcers, infection, mobility status, knowledge of diabetes
2. List the nursing diagnoses that would be applicable to Mrs. James' assessment.
   Infection, high risk for. Skin integrity, impaired, high risk for; physical mobility, impaired; body image disturbance; impaired vision
3. Describe the complications for which Mrs. James is at risk.
   Infection, pressure ulcers, trauma/injury
4. Describe nursing interventions for preventing the complications.
   Teach Mrs. James self care to prevent infections and skin injury, including foot care.
   Teach Mrs. James to do skin inspections routinely.
   Do diabetic teaching to avoid blood sugar imbalances.
   Evaluate home setting for potential dangers that could cause injury.

5. What specific actions would you take to prevent a recurrence of venous stasis ulcers?
   Assess other lower extremity for skin texture, color, edema, ulcerations, pain, calf tenderness. Encourage Mrs. James to elevate legs periodically throughout the day and to wear compression stocking if ordered by physician. Mrs. James should avoid use of round garters, monitor condition of her foot, wash and dry feet thoroughly, use moisturizing lotion.

6. What additional community services does Mrs. James need?
   Homemaker to do routine household chores.
   Meals-on-Wheels requesting diabetic meals.
   Make arrangements for podiatrist to provide foot and toenail care.

7. What nursing services would you plan to meet her needs; frequency of nurse visits, services from a nursing assistant, other home health services. Which services would each person provide?
   Home health nurse to do daily blood glucose checks and draw up insulin if Mrs. James' vision is too impaired for her to do this safely herself. Allow her to self-inject insulin. Home health nurse can continue and reinforce the teaching, do skin inspections. Home health aide to provide personal care several times a week.

8. Describe the outcomes you would expect for Mrs. James.
   Blood glucose level remains within acceptable parameters.
   Free of complications.
   Increasing independence in activities of daily living.

ANSWERS TO THE REVIEW QUESTIONS

1. One reason for the growth in non-acute care health services is:
   c. the cost of acute care.
2. Medicare is a reimbursement system for health care providers that:
   b. is available to persons 65 years of age and over or who have been disabled for two or more years.
3. Subacute care is most often provided:
   b. in a special care unit of a skilled care facility.
4. Which of the following clients would be most likely to benefit from rehabilitation services?
   a. Mr. J, sixty-four years old, who has had a stroke, is responsive and stable.
5. Which of the following is a legal requirement for health care facilities that is controlled by each state?
   c. Licensure
6. As a member of the interdisciplinary health care team, the LP/VN must be able to:
   a. participate in the planning of client care.
7. In the home health care setting it is essential that the LP/VN possess skills in:
   c. physical assessment.
8. In a long-term care facility the LP/VN may serve as the:
   a. charge nurse of a unit.

CHAPTER 18
The Dying Process/Hospice Care

SUGGESTED RESPONSES TO THE CASE STUDY

Mrs. Jason is seventy-six years old with a history of heart failure. She has been hospitalized twice within the last year and was critically ill both times. Both times she was discharged to her home. A home health nurse and a nursing assistant make intermittent visits to monitor her condition and to help with her activities of daily living. Her husband manages the household chores. Mrs. Jason's condition is deteriorating as the shortness of breath becomes more severe. Her energy level is easily depleted and it is getting more difficult for her to get out of bed. The family is concerned because Mrs. Jason does not have any advance directives. Any attempt to bring up the subject is met with avoidance and a change of subject.

1. List the clinical manifestations you would expect Mrs. Jason to experience.
   Dyspnea, edema, fatigue, increased heart rate, dysrhythmias, orthopnea.

2. Identify four nursing diagnoses to utilize in planning her care.
   (1) Cardiac output, decreased, related to ineffective pumping of heart
   (2) Fluid volume excess, related to low cardiac output
   (3) Activity intolerance, related to altered oxygen delivery to body tissues
   (4) Fear, related to deteriorating physical condition

3. Describe several nursing interventions for implementing palliative care.
   Administer medications to alleviate edema and to regulate heart beat.
   Position for comfort to ease breathing.
   Avoid rushing: give ample time and provide as much assistance as she needs, alternate periods of rest and activity, allow her to determine on which activities she wishes to expend her limited energy resources. Listen to her concerns; listen for "unspoken" messages.

4. Describe appropriate interactions with the family to ease their concerns.
   Provide information on the legalities of the state in which they reside, regarding their options in the event that Mrs. Jason dies without advance directives. Assure them that you will serve as an advocate for Mrs. Jason and the family.

5. Explain why you think Mrs. Jason and her family could benefit from hospice services.
   Hospice services could provide an individual who is experienced in working with Mrs. Jason and her fear.

ANSWERS TO THE REVIEW QUESTIONS

1. Anticipatory grieving is a process of:
   b. acknowledging impending death.
2. The purpose of the Patient Self-Determination Act is to:
   c. provide an opportunity for making one's wishes known in the event the client is unable to voice his/her wishes.
3. The basic premise of supportive care is to:
   b. provide emotional, physical, and mental comfort.
4. The hospice philosophy of care believes in:
   a. pain and symptom control.
5. Signs of impending death include:
   c. Cheyne-Stokes respirations.

CHAPTER 19

Respiratory Disorders

SUGGESTED RESPONSES TO THE CASE STUDY

Mrs. White is a seventy-seven-year-old female with a history of smoking two to three packs of cigarettes a day for the last 60 years. Mrs. White has been diagnosed with COPD for the past four years. She has required supplemental oxygen at 2 liters/min. for the last 18 months. Three days ago Mrs. White was admitted with a chief complaint of increasing dyspnea on exertion and a productive cough of thick green-yellow sputum. She states that she does not know why she is coughing up this awful stuff.

Physical examination of Mrs. White this morning revealed: vital signs of T = 101.5° F, P = 124, R = 38, BP = 168/74; sonorous and sibilant wheezes upon expiration in the posterior lung fields with superimposed coarse crackles heard in the right posterior lower lung field. She is unable to ambulate to the bathroom or complete other ADLs due to the dyspnea. Chest x-ray showed a large area of consolidation in the right lower lobe. Sputum culture is still pending.

1. List the clinical manifestations which indicate Mrs. White is experiencing an infection concomitant with her COPD.
    Increasing dyspnea on exertion; productive cough of thick, green-yellow sputum; sibilant and sonorous expiratory wheezes with coarse crackles; temperature 101.5°F; respiratory rate of 38; pulse rate 124 and consolidation of the right lung on chest X-ray.

2. Explain why COPD predisposes a client to respiratory infection.
    COPD results in an increase in the amount of respiratory secretions which provide a growth media for invading organisms.

3. Explain why the physician will increase Mrs. White's oxygen flow to 3–4 liters/minute.
    The physician will increase Mrs. White's oxygen to 3–4 liters/minute to maintain an oxygen saturation of 95 percent or greater. However, the increase in flow rate will be done cautiously as Mrs. White may have an altered respiratory drive that responds to lower levels of oxygen in the blood rather than higher levels of carbon dioxide.

4. List the subjective and objective data the nurse should obtain during the nursing assessment.
    Subjective: complaints of cough, dyspnea, fatigue; past medical history; smoking history.
    Objective: vital signs, respiratory effort, color, breath sounds, position assumed for ease of respiration; sputum production.

5. Write three nursing diagnoses and client goals which would be pertinent to Mrs. White's care.
    Nursing Diagnoses:
    (1) Activity intolerance related to hypoxia
    (2) Knowledge deficit related to signs and symptoms of respiratory infection
    (3) Gas exchange, impaired, related to disease processes
    Goals:
    (1) Mrs. White will exercise and increase activity within respiratory limitations.
    (2) Mrs. White will state signs and symptoms of a respiratory infection.
    (3) Mrs. White will have adequate gas exchange.

6. Prioritize the above diagnoses with the first being the highest priority.
    (1) Gas exchange, impaired, related to disease processes
    (2) Activity intolerance, related to hypoxia
    (3) Knowledge deficit, related to signs and symptoms of respiratory infection.

7. Describe client outcomes which would indicate Mrs. White's treatment and nursing care regimen are successful.

Mrs. White will have a respiratory rate, color, respiratory effort, and oxygen saturation within normal limits. Mrs. White is able to carry out prescribed activities without dyspnea. Mrs. White is able to identify signs and symptoms of respiratory infection from a list.

ANSWERS TO THE REVIEW QUESTIONS

1. The physician orders oxygen to be delivered to the client with COPD at 2–3 liters because:
   c. a higher flow rate may suppress the client's drive to breathe.
2. A particulate respirator mask is used by the nurse caring for a client with tuberculosis because:
   a. regular masks allow the tubercle bacilli to pass through.
3. Bronchodilators are used to treat bronchiectasis in order to:
   b. dilate airways that have lost their elasticity.
4. Incentive spirometry is used to measure the amount of air that:
   c. is inspired with one inhalation.
5. Asthma is characterized by:
   b. intermittent airflow obstruction.
6. The client with a pneumothorax experiences hypoxia due to:
   b. compression of the lung tissue underlying the pneumothorax.

CHAPTER 20
Cardiac Disorders

SUGGESTED RESPONSES TO THE CASE STUDY

Mr. Lance Jeffers, a fifty-five-year-old truck driver, was admitted to the emergency room with a feeling of heavy squeezing pressure in his sternal area. The pain is radiating to his left shoulder. He is diaphoretic, short of breath, and nauseated. He states the sternal pain came on suddenly while watching a football game. He had been mowing his yard and decided to rest. The emergency physician gives Mr. Jeffers a nitroglycerin tablet and connects him to an EKG monitor. Cardiac enzymes with isoenzyme fractions and a chest x-ray are requested STAT. Morphine sulfate 2 mg is given intravenously. The EKG shows no Q waves, a depressed ST wave, and T wave changes. Oxygen is given by mask at 4 liters/minute. Mr. Jeffers' apical pulse is 102 and his blood pressure is 130/88. A cardiac catheterization with fluoroscopy is ordered to determine the patency of the coronary blood vessels and functioning of the heart muscle. Three hours after admission, crackles are heard in the lungs, the $CK_2(MB)$ is elevated, and the LDH_1 is higher than the LDH_2.

1. List symptoms/clinical manifestations, other than Mr. Jeffers', a client may experience when having a myocardial infarction.

   Other symptoms a client may experience when having a myocardial infarction are: anxiousness; vomiting; irregular, rapid, and weak pulse; hypotension; skin pale or cyanotic.

2. List two reasons morphine sulfate was given to Mr. Jeffers.

   Morphine sulfate relieves pain (analgesic effect), decreases anxiety, slows respirations, relaxes bronchial smooth muscles allowing a better exchange of oxygen and carbon dioxide. It causes

blood to pool in the peripheries rather than returning to the heart and lungs, thus decreasing the workload of the heart.

3.   List two other diagnostic tests that may have been ordered for Mr. Jeffers.

Other diagnostic tests that may have been ordered for Mr. Jeffers are radioactive isotope scan, myocardial scintigraphy, MUGA, CBC, and erythrocyte sedimentation rate.

4.   List subjective and objective data a nurse would want to obtain about Mr. Jeffers.

Subjective data: Medications Mr. Jeffers has taken including over-the-counter medications, anti-coagulants, and thrombolytic medications. Assess Mr. Jeffer's pain as to onset, duration, intensity, location, radiation, and precipitating factors. Ask Mr. Jeffers to describe his symptoms in detail. Inquire as to Mr. Jeffers' ability to perform activities of daily living.

Objective data: Monitor the vital signs for an irregular, decreased, or increased pulse or a decreased or elevated blood pressure. Watch for pallor, cyanosis, diaphoresis, or vomiting. Assess for cool clammy skin, numbness, tingling, or confusion which would indicate decreased oxygenation of the tissues. Listen to the breath sounds for lung congestion. Monitor the EKG for dysrhythmias. Notice if Mr. Jeffers is grimacing, clenching his hands, or clutching his chest. Watch closely for these symptoms as activities are increased.

5.   Write three individualized nursing diagnoses and goals for Mr. Jeffers.

Possible nursing diagnoses include:

(1) Cardiac output, decreased, related to damaged heart tissue

(2) Pain, acute, chest, related to decreased oxygenation of myocardial tissue

(3) Anxiety, moderate, related to concern about disease process and future socioeconomic status

(4) Activity intolerance, related to decreased circulation to body tissues.

(5) Constipation, high risk for, related to opiate analgesics and bed rest

(6) Knowledge deficit, related to disease process, medications, diet, and plan for recovery

Possible goals for Mr. Jeffers are:

(1) Mr. Jeffers will have increased cardiac output.

(2) Mr. Jeffers will verbalize decrease in frequency and intensity of chest pain.

(3) Mr. Jeffers will verbalize situations that are causing stress.

(4) Mr. Jeffers will increase activities with decreased symptoms of angina, dyspnea, cyanosis, and dysrhythmia.

(5) Mr. Jeffers will have soft bowel movements.

(6) Mr. Jeffers will verbalize understanding of disease process, diet, activity, and medications.

6.   Mr. Jeffers is moved from the critical care unit. List pertinent nursing actions a nurse would do in caring for Mr. Jeffers related to:

oxygenation	activity
cardiac output	medications
comfort/rest	teaching

Nursing interventions related to oxygenation: Oxygen will be given per mask or nasal cannula at 2–4 liters per minute.

Nursing interventions related to cardiac output: Mr. Jeffers would be placed on bed rest until his condition is stabilized.

An IV will be started so medications such as morphine and antidysrhythmics can be administered. If beta blockers are administered, the nurse should closely monitor for a drop in heart rate and blood pressure. Constantly monitor Mr. Jeffers for dysrhythmias. A rhythm strip is placed on the chart at least once a shift. Three dysrhythmias that may occur following an MI are ventricular fibrillation, bradycardias, and tachycardias. Ventricular fibrillation is treated by defibrillation. Atropine and, if needed, a temporary pacer may be inserted for bradycardias. Two tachycardias that may occur are atrial fibrillation and ventricular tachycardia. Atrial fibrillation is treated with digoxin (Lanoxin) or amiodarone (Cordarone). Ventricular tachycardia is treated with lidocaine or cardioversion. If dysrhythmias continue, magnesium may be given. Administer medications as prescribed by the physician.

Nursing interventions related to comfort/rest: Place objects within reach of the client. Balance activity with rest periods. Mr. Jeffers and his family are encouraged to verbalize their feelings. Provide a quiet, calm environment to help Mr. Jeffers and his family relax. Mr. Jeffers should be provided periods of uninterrupted rest.

Nursing interventions related to activity: Place objects within reach of the client. Balance activity with rest periods. Before Mr. Jeffers is dismissed, low-intensity exercise tests may be done to determine the types of activities Mr. Jeffers may engage in at home.

Nursing interventions related to medications: Administer medications as prescribed by the physician. Sedatives may be given to help the client relax. Teach Mr. Jeffers about the actions, dosage times, and side effects of medications he is taking.

Nursing interventions related to teaching: Mr. Jeffers is instructed to inform the nurse of any chest pain or shortness of breath. Teach Mr. Jeffers about the anatomy and physiology of the heart, what physiologically happened to his heart to cause the myocardial infarction, importance of exercise, diet instructions, actions and side effects of medications, importance of not smoking, and stress reduction. When Mr. Jeffers is able to climb two flights of stairs, sexual activity may be resumed. Discuss Mr. Jeffers and his wife's fears and feelings candidly.

7. List resources specific to locale that could assist Mr. Jeffers in his cardiac rehabilitation.
   Refer Mr. Jeffers to the American Heart Association or Mended Hearts, Inc. or other resources specific to locale.

8. List teachings that Mr. Jeffers will need before his discharge.
   Refer to teaching under question 6 for suggestions on discharge teaching.

9. List at least three successful client outcomes for Mr. Jeffers.
   (1) Mr. Jeffers will have increased cardiac output as manifested by decreased dyspnea, improved temperature in lower extremities, improved pedal pulses.
   (2) Mr. Jeffers will verbalize decrease in frequency and intensity of chest pain.
   (3) Mr. Jeffers will increase activities with decreased symptoms of angina, dyspnea, cyanosis, and dysrhythmia.
   (4) Mr. Jeffers will verbalize situations that are causing stress and practice stress reduction techniques.
   (5) Mr. Jeffers will have soft bowel movements by increasing fiber in his diet and drinking adequate liquids.
   (6) Mr. Jeffers will explain his disease process, diet, activity limitations, and medications.

ANSWERS TO THE REVIEW QUESTIONS

1. The volume of blood pumped by the left ventricle per minute is:
   b. cardiac output.
2. A coronary artery disease risk factor that can be modified or altered is:
   c. stress.
3. The nurse may assist in relieving the chest pain of a client with pericarditis by having the client:
   d. sit erect and lean forward.
4. To assess a client with right-sided heart failure, the nurse would:
   c. check for distended neck veins with the bed at a 45° angle.
5. A diagnostic test for a myocardial infarction is:
   a. cardiac enzymes.
6. It would be important to teach a client with angina to
   b. carry nitroglycerin tablets at all times.
7. A client with the diagnosis of a myocardial infarction has just been admitted to the ER. To relieve chest pain the physician orders:
   d. morphine sulfate.
8. A cardiac dysrhythmia that has an erratic electrical activity of the atria resulting in a rate of 350 beats/minute to 600 beats/minute is:
   a. atrial fibrillation.
9. A nursing intervention to improve cardiac output is:
   d. administer oxygen per physician orders.
10. The most appropriate nursing diagnosis for a client with coronary artery disease is:
    a. decreased cardiac output.

CHAPTER 21

Vascular Disorders

SUGGESTED RESPONSES TO THE CASE STUDY

> *Lucille Soudin, a sixty-three-year-old female, slipped on a throw rug in her home and fell. She immediately had severe pain in her right hip. Her husband called the emergency service, and she was transferred to the local hospital. Lucille was admitted to the hospital and scheduled for a total hip replacement.*
>
> *In the evening of the first postoperative day, Lucille stated the calf of her right leg was "hurting." The nurse placed her hand on the area where Lucille indicated there was pain and found the posterior area of the right calf to be warm, reddened, and tender to touch.*

1. What other assessments should the nurse make before calling the physician?
   The nurse obtains vital signs and checks the leg for hardness along the involved vessel, unilateral edema, superficial vein dilation, and leg heaviness or tightness. Ask if Mrs. Soudin has had any chest pain, dyspnea, tachycardia, or hemoptysis.

2. Should the nurse perform a Homan's sign at this time?
   No. Performing the Homan's sign may dislodge the clot.

3. What orders may the nurse receive from the physician?
   The physician may give orders for bed rest, warm soaks to the affected area, elevation of extremity with the knee slightly flexed and legs supported with pillows, circumference of affected leg measured every eight hours, peripheral pulse taken every four hours, observation for signs of occlusion such as absence of pulse, pallor, pain, and coldness to extremity and elastic support hose. The nurse may also receive an order for heparin.

4. What medications may have been ordered prophylactically to prevent a thrombus formation? What baseline laboratory results should be obtained before the anticoagulant medications are started?
   Heparin or enoxaparin sodium injection (Lovenox), a low-molecular-weight heparin, are used prophylactically.
   A PTT or APTT would be ordered before the heparin is given and a PT or INR is done before Coumadin is started. A CBC and platelet count are monitored throughout Lovenox therapy.

5. Write pertinent individualized nursing diagnoses and goals for Lucille.
   Nursing diagnoses:
   (1) Tissue perfusion, altered, peripheral, related to decreased blood flow and possible clot formation
   (2) Pain, related to decreased circulation in lower extremity secondary to thrombi
   (3) Anxiety, related to possibility of the clot becoming an embolus
   (4) Knowledge deficit, related to disease process and risk factors
   Goals:
   (1) Lucille will have no symptoms of clot formation.
   (2) Lucille will state absence of pain.
   (3) Lucille will verbalize concern of clot complications.
   (4) Lucille will list measures to prevent thrombus formation.

6. List appropriate nursing interventions needed in providing care to Lucille. (Refer also to Chapter 26, Musculoskeletal Disorders, for total hip replacement postop care.)
   (1) Tissue perfusion, altered, peripheral: Lucille's entire affected leg should be elevated when on bed rest to improve venous return. When elevated, the leg is slightly flexed at the knee with a pillow under the thigh and calf. Elastic support stockings are worn. If anticoagulant drugs are given, assess for signs of bleeding which include hematuria, bruising, bleeding from the

gums, and blood in the stool. Observe for symptoms of clot formation in the groin and if there are symptoms notify the physician.

(2) **Pain:** Encourage active range of motion (ROM) exercises with the unaffected leg while the client is on bed rest or relatively inactive. Apply warm moist soaks to the affected area. Administer analgesics as ordered for discomfort. Teach Lucille how to use the overhead trapeze bar to assist in moving in bed. Maintain proper alignment in bed. Check the incision site frequently and observe for signs of infection. Place pillows or a splint between Lucille's legs when turning her.

(3) **Anxiety:** Encourage Lucille to verbalize her concern of a clot becoming an embolus. Instruct Lucille of the importance of maintaining bed rest so as not to dislodge the clot. By informing Lucille of the importance of bed rest, she will have a participatory role in her care and decrease her anxiety level.

(4) **Knowledge deficit:** Before discharge, instruct the client to drink 2–3 quarts of water per day, not to sit with legs crossed, elevate her legs when sitting, avoid sitting or standing for extended periods, and to wear support hose. If Lucille experiences leg pain, tenderness, or swelling, difficulty breathing, or chest pain, the physician should be notified immediately. If Lucille is discharged on anticoagulant therapy, instruct her to take the medication at the same time each day, maintain appointments to have the PT or INR level checked, watch for signs of bleeding, and avoid aspirin or medications containing aspirin. Aspirin increases the clotting time. Notify the physician if abdominal pain occurs.

7. What information should the nurse include in Lucille's discharge teaching regarding:
   symptoms of another thrombus: **If the client experiences leg pain, tenderness or swelling, difficulty breathing or chest pain, the physician should be notified immediately.**
   anticoagulant therapy: **If on anticoagulant therapy, instruct the client to take the medication at the same time each day, maintain appointments to have the PT or INR level checked, watch for signs of bleeding, and avoid aspirin or drugs containing aspirin. Aspirin increases the clotting time. A physician should be notified if abdominal pain occurs, as this could indicate internal bleeding.**
   elevation and positioning of the extremity: **Because of the total hip replacement surgery, Lucille should not cross her legs or sit with her knees higher than her hips.**

8. List resources specific to locale that could assist in Lucille's rehabilitation process.
   If Lucille's husband is not able to care for her after discharge, a transitional care facility may assist with care. Possibly her husband could care for her at home with assistance from a home care facility. Local outpatient rehabilitation or physical therapy facilities may assist with outpatient therapy needs. (These facilities should be located within the student's locale.)

9. List successful client outcomes for Lucille.
   (1) **Lucille has had no symptoms of clot formation.**
   (2) **Lucille was able to control the pain with prescribed analgesics.**
   (3) **Lucille is expressing concerns regarding clot complications.**
   (4) **Lucille listed measures to prevent thrombus formation before discharge.**

ANSWERS TO THE REVIEW QUESTIONS

1. The valves are a part of which tunica layer?
   a. tunica intima
2. A test that a nurse performs to evaluate the arterial circulation of the hands is the:
   c. Allen's test.
3. Instructions to a client on anticoagulant therapy includes:
   b. watching for symptoms of bleeding.
4. When assessing a client with a possible DVT, the nurse:
   c. gently touches the affected area and checks for warmth.
5. A varicose vein is more likely to occur in the:
   d. saphenous vein.
6. A nurse is assigned to care for a client who has just had a hysterectomy. To prevent the formation of a thrombus, the nurse:
   b. encourages the client to ambulate with assistance according to the physician's orders.

7. A client, admitted with the diagnosis of AAA, states he can feel a pulsation when he lies flat in bed. To assess the pulsation, the nurse would palpate:
   d. left of umbilicus.
8. The symptoms a client would most likely experience who has an aneurysm pressing on the inferior vena cava would be:
   d. edema in the extremities and possible cyanosis.
9. The first step of the stepped-care approach in treating hypertension is:
   a. changes in lifestyle.
10. A thirty-two-year-old client has a pulse rate of 72. When she exercises her target heart rate is:
   c. 141.

CHAPTER 22
Blood and Lymph Disorders

SUGGESTED RESPONSES TO THE CASE STUDY

James Johns, forty-six, owns a hobby shop. He has had a cold for three weeks that has recently settled in his chest. He has been tired lately and takes naps each evening before the evening meal. His wife noticed several bruises on his arms and legs but James could not recall any particular injury. James has gradually lost 10 pounds over the last three months but has not been concerned about it. When James went to the clinic for some antibiotics for his cold, the nurse practitioner completed a physical assessment and ordered a chest x-ray and CBC. The nurse practitioner noticed the WBCs were 250,000/mm^3, RBCs 4.2 million/ mm^3 and the platelets were 100,000/mm^3. After several other tests were performed over the next few days, a diagnosis of CML was confirmed.

1. List the symptoms occurring in James Johns that are typical of CML.
   James Johns may be exposed to benzene, found in airplane glue, in his hobby shop. CML often manifests itself as an infection such as pneumonia. Other symptoms of CML James manifested were fatigue, bruising, and weight loss.

2. List five other typical symptoms of CML that were not stated in the case study.
   Other typical symptoms of CML are fever, chills, pallor, malaise, tachycardia, tachypnea, petechiae, bruising, epistaxis, melena, gingival bleeding, increased menstrual bleeding, night sweats, swollen lymph nodes, headaches, visual disturbances, and pain.

3. List other diagnostic tests to confirm the diagnosis of CML.
   Besides the CBC, other diagnostic tests to confirm the diagnosis of CML are bone marrow biopsy and Philadelphia chromosome (Ph^1).

4. List subjective and objective data the nurse practitioner would obtain about James Johns.
   To obtain subjective data, the nurse would ask about previous symptoms the client has experienced; familial history of chromosomal abnormalities; history of exposure to chemicals, viral infections, and previous chemotherapy or radiation therapy; presence of any pain (location, type, and duration); symptoms of infection (cough, pain, or burning on urination); a history of bleeding such as epistaxis, gingival bleeding, melena, or hematuria.

   To obtain objective data, the nurse assesses for signs of infection and bleeding. Common sites for infection include the mouth, pharynx, lungs, skin, bladder, and perianal area. Assessment for bleeding includes monitoring the platelet count, as bleeding occurs easily if the platelet count falls below 50,000. Clients can bleed from any orifice, so it is important for the nurse to inspect any discharge from the body.

5. Write three individualized nursing diagnoses and goals for James Johns.

    Individualized nursing diagnoses for James Johns include:

    Knowledge deficit, related to disease process and treatment as manifested by lack of knowledge about CML.

    Infection, related to increased production of immature white blood cells as manifested by pneumonia.

    Injury, high risk for, related to decreased production of platelets.

    Activity intolerance, related to decreased energy sources from disease process as manifested by fatigue and taking naps before evening meal.

    Nutrition, altered, less than body requirements, related to effects of disease process as manifested by loss of 10 pounds over last three months

    Goals for James Johns include:

    The client will: relate treatment methods and possible complications of chemotherapy; list signs and symptoms of infection; identify ways to avoid injury and prevent bleeding; list ways to conserve energy; choose nonirritating, high-protein, high-carbohydrate meals and snacks.

6. List nursing interventions for James Johns.

    Knowledge deficit: Teach the client to observe for signs of infection and bleeding. Review side effects of chemotherapy and radiation with James Johns and his wife.

    Infection: Explain the importance of good hand-washing techniques to James' family and friends who come in contact with him. Encourage James to use antimicrobial soaps for his daily bath. Teach James the importance of frequent oral care with a soft toothbrush and nonirritating mouthwash to prevent open sores and stomatitis. Teach James to cleanse the perianal area after each bowel movement to decrease bacterial contamination and prevent rectal fissures. Avoid rectal temperatures and suppositories. Take James' temperature every four hours to monitor for signs of infection. Report any temperature over 100°F to the nurse practitioner. Teach James to notify the nurse practitioner any time his temperature is over 100°F. Administer antibiotics and antifungals as ordered. Monitor respiration rates and breath sounds closely.

    Bleeding: Observe James for signs of bleeding such as confusion, epistaxis, gingival bleeding, petechiae, ecchymosis, hematemesis, enlarged abdomen, hematuria, and melena. Administer stool softeners as needed. Use cotton swabs instead of a toothbrush for oral care. Encourage James to use an electric razor. Avoid giving injections as much as possible. If a catheter is needed, lubricate it well to avoid trauma to the mucosal lining of the urethra.

    Activity intolerance: Teach James to plan daily activities so there is a balance of exercise and rest.

    Nutrition altered: Have a dietitian instruct James and his wife about a high-protein, high-carbohydrate diet to prevent infection and provide needed energy. Supplement the diet with vitamins. Teach James to avoid raw fruits and vegetables as these foods may contain more bacteria than cooked foods.

7. List community resources specific to locale that could assist James and his family during his illness with CML.

    Local community resources could include cancer or leukemia support groups, hospice, or visiting nurse service.

8. List discharge teaching the nurse would give to James and his family.

    Teach the client to observe for signs of infection and bleeding. Teach James to notify the nurse practitioner any time his temperature is over 100°F.

9. List successful client outcomes for James Johns.

    James will: relate treatment methods and possible complications of chemotherapy by discharge; list signs and symptoms of infection by discharge; identify ways to avoid injury and prevent bleeding by time of discharge; plan daily activities so there is a balance of activity and rest; list foods high in protein and carbohydrate by time of discharge.

10. List chemotherapeutic agents and side effects of the agents that may be prescribed for James.

    Chemotherapy agents for CML include busulfan (Myleran), hydroxyurea and DAT (daunorubicin HCl, ara-C, thioguanine). Complications of chemotherapy are nausea, vomiting, and stomatitis. Alopecia occurs 1–2 weeks after treatments are initiated. During chemotherapy the reduced white cell count may stop the formation of pus so infection may instead manifest as redness, swelling, and pain.

11. List other medical treatments that may be ordered for James.

    In the CML chronic phase, HLA-identical allogenic bone marrow is given and the client's own treated bone marrow is given in the blastic phase.

12. What measures could the nurse take to meet the emotional needs of James and his family?

    A nurse on each shift could set aside ten minutes to talk with James and his family. The nurse encourages the client to voice his concerns and fears related to having leukemia. The nurse makes referrals to support groups, social workers, and clergy as needed.

ANSWERS TO THE REVIEW QUESTIONS

1. The diagnostic test for sickle cell anemia is the:

   c. hemoglobin electrophoresis.

2. For improved iron absorption, a client with iron deficiency anemia takes Feosol with:

   b. an orange.

3. A thorough assessment of the cardiac system on a client with sickle cell anemia is important because:

   a. the heart enlarges in an attempt to provide the oxygen needs to the body tissues.

4. Clients with leukemia are prone to infections because:

   d. the WBCs are incapable of fighting infections.

5. To treat a leukemic client who has symptoms of a headache and visual disturbances, the physician may order:

   d. Methotrexate intrathecally.

6. A nursing action for a client with pernicious anemia is to:

   b. administer cyanocobalamin (vitamin B$_{12}$) as ordered.

7. Nursing care for a client with polycythemia vera includes:

   a. doing a Homan's sign to check for blood clots.

8. Symptoms that alert a nurse that a client may have DIC are:

   c. purpura, bruising, and decreased urine output.

9. A client with hemophilia is taught to:

   a. administer clotting factors as needed.

10. Encourage a client with non-Hodgkin's lymphoma to

    d. avoid exposure to infections.

CHAPTER 23

Integumentary Disorders

SUGGESTED RESPONSES TO THE CASE STUDY

Maude Murphy, age sixty-eight, noticed that the skin on the outside of her left lower leg just above the ankle was changing in color and texture. The skin felt rigid and didn't move as easily as skin on the upper part of her leg did. Itching was becoming a problem. Inadvertently she would scratch the area, sometimes causing small excoriations. One day she bumped her leg against the rough edge of the outside steps as she was going into the house. The cut was only an inch long and wasn't very deep. Over the next few weeks she noticed that instead of healing, it was getting bigger and was becoming quite painful. The skin around the wound was red and swollen. The yellow drainage coming from the wound had a bad smell. She had never had this kind of problem before. She did have varicose veins in that leg, and while she knew that she was uncomfortable if she was standing for long periods, she didn't think the problem was serious. When she went to the doctor, he diagnosed a venous stasis ulcer and cultured the drainage. He ordered the following treatment:

1. *Cefaclor (Ceclor) 500 mg p.o. every 8 hours for two weeks.*
2. *Wet-to-dry dressings with normal saline solution. Change every 8 hours.*
3. *Bed rest with left leg elevated. May have bathroom privileges and be up for meals.*

The doctor explained that he would be ordering an Unna's boot after the wound was debrided and the infection controlled so that she could be ambulatory, but that even after the Unna's boot was applied, he would want her to have rest periods during the day with her leg elevated. Mrs. Murphy thought she could learn to change the dressings, but she expressed doubt that she could stay in bed most of the time. She was used to being up and active and getting her work done each day.

1. List the clinical manifestations of a venous stasis ulcer.
   With impaired circulation, the skin of the lower leg gradually loses resilient subcutaneous tissue. The skin hardens and becomes dark red to brown in color. This tissue is easily injured and heals very slowly because of the impaired circulation. Itching accompanies these changes in skin texture. Venous stasis ulcers begin as small, tender inflamed areas above the ankle. A slight trauma causes an open area that does not heal, but instead gradually worsens to a shallow ulcer. The ulcer becomes painful. Infection is common, causing a foul-smelling drainage. The center of the ulcer may have strands of yellow fibrous tissue. Edema surrounds the ulcer.

2. What is the usual medical treatment?
   Usual medical treatment includes: antibiotics to treat the infection; enzyme preparations or normal saline wet-to-dry dressings to debride the ulcer of necrotic tissue; elevation of the extremity above the level of the heart, sharply limiting the amount of time standing or sitting with the leg dependent; and with small, non-infected ulcers, use of an Unna's boot to provide support during ambulation and to prevent stasis of venous blood.

3. List the subjective and objective assessment data that the nurse should obtain from Maude Murphy.
   Subjective data: How long has the ulcer been present? Describe the pain. What kind of pain? What is the duration? Rate the pain on a scale of 0 to 10. What helps relieve the pain? Does the skin around the ulcer itch? Does the client scratch it? What helps relieve the itching? What is Maude's mobility and dexterity status? Can she reach the ulcer? Can she apply medications and dressings without contaminating the open wound?
   Objective data: Describe the location of the ulcer and the appearance of the ulcer. What does the tissue look like? What is the color? Measure the size of the ulcer. Is there any drainage from the ulcer? Describe the amount, appearance, and odor of the drainage. Describe the appearance of the tissue surrounding the ulcer. Is there any pitting edema? If so, where? How much? Describe the color of the tissue. Is there a difference in color in the leg and ulcer when the client is lying down with the leg extended compared to when the client is sitting with the leg in a dependent position? Check for posterior tibial and dorsalis pedis pulses.

4. Write two to four individualized nursing diagnoses to address these problems.
   Appropriate nursing diagnoses include:
   (1) Tissue perfusion, altered, peripheral, related to edema and venous stasis as evidenced by swelling, itching, inflammation, and erythema.
   (2) Pain, chronic, related to tissue trauma and inflammation as evidenced by Maude's description of pain and itching.
   (3) Management of therapeutic regimen, individual, ineffective, related to Maude's questioning the seriousness of the problem as evidenced by her doubting that she could remain on bed rest.
   (4) Home maintenance management, impaired, related to a change in functional ability as evidenced by the pain of the ulcer, the need for bed rest, and Maude's expressed doubts of being able to stay in bed.
   Students might also identify the following nursing diagnoses, all of which are possible, but none of which are validated as actual nursing diagnoses by the data presented in the case study.

(5) **Risk for diversional activity deficit, related to prescribed bed rest and the inability to carry out usual activities**

(6) **Risk for hopelessness, related to continued pain, prolonged activity restrictions, and slow healing**

(7) **Risk for individual coping, ineffective, related to stress of a chronic condition with long-term treatment requirements**

(8) **Risk for body image disturbance, related to changes in physical appearance and ability to carry out daily activities**

Maude already has an infection in the ulcer that is being treated with antibiotics, so high risk for infection is not an appropriate nursing diagnosis to develop at this time. Altered physical mobility is not appropriate. Maude does not have the major defining characteristics of impaired physical mobility. Neither does Maude have the major defining characteristics for a nursing diagnosis of activity intolerance.

5. What will be the goals (expected outcomes) of nursing treatment?

(1) **Client will follow prescribed regimen and exhibit signs of improved circulation in lower extremities.**

(2) **Client will adhere to treatment recommendations and report a decrease in pain level.**

(3) **Client will describe possible complications of untreated venous stasis ulcers and follow prescribed activity restrictions.**

(4) **Client will limit activities to self care and explore possible sources of short-term household help.**

6. List appropriate nursing actions for each diagnosis. Include basic nursing care measures. Be specific about client education needs. Address nutrition and pharmacologic implications. Give a rationale for each action. **Measures are listed by order of diagnosis. Rationale appears in parentheses following the measure.**

(1) **Keep left leg elevated above the level of the heart when in bed or chair. (Prevents venous stasis. Improves venous blood flow. Helps decrease edema. As a result, cellular nutrition and oxygenation are improved.)**

   Do not sit with legs crossed. Do not wear garters or girdles. (Crossing legs and wearing restrictive garments impedes blood flow.)

   Change positions. Wiggle toes. Dorsiflex and plantar flex feet six to eight times each hour. (Muscle contractions assist circulation by moving blood from superficial veins to deeper veins, thus preventing venous stasis and pooling.)

(2) **Keep left leg elevated. (Edema increases pain in the ulcer. Elevating the extremity helps decrease edema.)**

   Take antibiotic every eight hours as prescribed. (As infection clears, inflammation and edema subside, thus relieving pain.)

   Follow physician's advice about taking a mild analgesic such as ibuprofen or acetaminophen 30 to 45 minutes before changing wet-to-dry dressings. (Changing the dressing after the onset of action of the medication will be less painful.)

(3) **Collaborate with the physician regarding referral to a home care nurse to make home visits to assess Maude's self-care abilities, give her guidance, reassure her, and assess her progress. (As Maude learns about her disease and becomes confident in her ability to care for herself, she is more likely to adhere to the treatment regimen.)**

   Limit time up for meal preparation to 30 minutes. Elevate left leg while sitting up to eat. (Prolonged standing increases venous pooling, stasis, and pain.)

   Discuss diet with Maude. She needs a balanced diet with increased vitamin C and protein for healing. Avoid foods high in sodium. Teach her to read labels to select foods. (Sodium can contribute to fluid retention. By reading labels, Maude can select foods that are low in sodium, but that have the balanced nutrients that she needs for wound healing.)

   Assist Maude to plan menus that are balanced yet require minimal preparation time. Suggest six small meals a day instead of three large ones. (She can meet her nutritional needs without prolonged standing while she prepares her meals. Small amounts of regularly planned activity may help decrease the boredom of inactivity.)

   Maintain a fluid intake of 2,000 to 2,500 mL daily. (This amount of fluid is a normal daily requirement. All cells must be adequately hydrated to function well.)

Explain to Maude how a venous stasis ulcer develops. Show her pictures and give her written information to refer to. Teach her to assess the appearance of the wound with each dressing change:

a. Look for signs of healing—wound base of red granulation tissue without yellow wound exudate; wound margins that have become well defined; size of the wound decreasing. The wound will heal by secondary intention; i.e., from the inside out.

b. Call the physician if any signs of infection are observed: increased pain and redness; increased amount of foul-smelling drainage; increased amount of yellow necrotic tissue in wound. (Involving Maude in her daily care enables her to monitor her progress and encourages her to follow the prescribed regimen. Understanding her condition and being involved in her care can contribute to her sense of self-control.)

(4) Encourage Maude to make a list of essential daily activities and a list of activities that can "wait a while." Review the list several times, making changes until the list of "essentials" is down to a few basic items. (This process of review and discussion helps to separate what one first "thinks" is essential from those things that really are "essential." Recognizing that she can get the "essentials" done will decrease Maude's frustration, thus encouraging compliance with the prescribed regimen.)

Explore with Maude viable options for obtaining some household help once or twice a week for a few weeks until the infection in the ulcer has cleared and the doctor can apply the Unna's boot, which will allow her to increase her activity. (Seeing that her house is in order will decrease Maude's anxiety about those things she thinks she needs to do, but knows that she should not do until the ulcer improves.)

7. Describe how to evaluate goal achievement for Maude Murphy.
(1) Is there evidence of improved circulation to the lower left leg? What is the appearance of the ulcer? What is the skin color? Have the edema, itching, and inflammation decreased?
(2) Does Maude describe decreased pain and discomfort?
(3) Has Maude taken her medication as prescribed? Has she changed the wet-to-dry dressings every eight hours? Did she limit her daily activity to meal preparation and bathroom privileges for hygiene and toileting? What is her assessment of her situation? How difficult was it for her to follow the plan of care? Can she describe how a venous stasis ulcer develops? Can she state the signs of healing? Of infection?
(4) How did she manage her day-to-day activities? Was she able to get some temporary help? How does she feel about her home situation? If the house and yard look less than "ideal," is it bothering her? What does she say?

ANSWERS TO THE REVIEW QUESTIONS

1. The skin has a vital role in the normal functioning of the human organism. That role is:
   b. protection from invasion by microorganisms.
2. The nurse charted that the client's skin was loose, wrinkled, and thin with mild scaling. The nurse was describing:
   b. texture.
3. An effective nursing intervention related to the care of open burn wounds that require daily dressing changes would be:
   c. Wear a cap, gown, mask, and sterile gloves when providing wound care.
4. The client has lesions on his scalp and on his arms near his elbows. The lesions appear as red patches covered with thick silvery scales. The most likely cause of these lesions is:
   c. psoriasis.
5. A nursing care plan for a client with an infectious disorder of the skin would include interventions to teach the client:
   a. how to avoid spreading the infection to others.
6. Which of the following is a malignant tumor?
   c. melanoma
7. Clients with pemphigus vulgaris often have a nutritional deficit. Which of the following nursing interventions can help improve the client's nutritional intake?
   c. Give mouth care with normal saline or a mild baking soda solution before meals.

CHAPTER 24

Allergies, Immune, and Autoimmune Disorders

SUGGESTED RESPONSES TO THE CASE STUDY

Sharon is a thirty-four-year-old divorced African American woman. Five years ago she was diagnosed with SLE. Recently, she developed a urinary tract infection that has not responded to medication. Yesterday, when she visited her physician, she complained that the pain in her hands and wrists is getting worse. She was admitted to the hospital for evaluation and rehabilitation.

Sharon has three children, ages 16, 12, and 8. Her husband divorced her several years ago. She tells you "He just couldn't take it anymore. He was working full time. When he came home he would have to do all the housework and care for the children." She now lives with her mother. Sharon used to work as an aide in a nursing home, but due to constant fatigue she had to quit.

Upon admission Sharon's vital signs were as follows: temperature 100.6°F, blood pressure 170/94, pulse 84, respirations 20. Physical exam revealed the presence of a butterfly rash. This is the first symptom she developed. She had hoped it would go away after she started taking prednisone (Meticorten) but it has remained. She relates that she does not go out in public anymore because everyone stares at her. The assessment revealed that the joints in her hands are stiff; she stated that she has difficulty using her fork.

Initial lab results are:

Urinalysis = Bacteria count greater than 100,000/milliliter
ESR = 24 mm/hr
RBCs = 3.2
WBCs = 15,035
LE Cell Test = Positive
Hemoglobin = 9.2
ANA = Positive

1. List signs and symptoms, other than those identified above, clients with SLE might experience.
   Fever, leukopenia, thrombocytopenia, anorexia, hypertension, respiratory and cardiac infections, renal involvement, irritability, confusion, hallucinations, enlarged liver, spleen photosensitivity, and irregular menses.

2. Since Sharon has a history of long-term use of corticosteroids, what side effects might she experience?
   Moon face, hypertension, hyperglycemia, hypernatremia, hypokalemia, muscle wasting, enlarged abdomen, and a buffalo hump.

3. What diagnostic tests might be ordered to evaluate her arthritic condition?
   RBCs, WBCs, platelet count, ESR, ANA, C-reactive protein, and RF

4. Write three nursing diagnoses and goals for Sharon.
   ***Nursing Diagnosis 1:* Physical mobility, impaired, related to pain, edema, and joint immobility as evidenced by difficulty using a fork.**
   ***Goal:* Sharon will implement methods to decrease joint pain and increase mobility.**
   ***Nursing Diagnosis 2:* Body image disturbance, related to butterfly rash as evidenced by reluctance to go out in public.**
   ***Goal:* Sharon will verbalize and demonstrate acceptance of appearance.**
   ***Nursing Diagnosis 3:* Fatigue, related to chronic inflammatory process, as evidenced by verbalization of being tired all the time.**
   ***Goal:* Sharon will balance daily activities with periods of rest.**

5. Identify nursing interventions to help Sharon deal with:

   Impaired mobility: While in the hospital, encourage Sharon to use the overhead trapeze when moving in bed. Check with physician about a referral to occupational and physical therapy. Teach Sharon to use assistive devices. Teach Sharon ROM exercises and encourage her to perform them several times each day.

   Joint pain: Instruct Sharon on action, duration, and side effects of prescribed analgesic medications. Teach Sharon relaxation techniques. Encourage Sharon to take a warm shower upon awakening.

   Fatigue: Allow Sharon time to express feelings about being tired all the time. Encourage Sharon to identify essential activities needed to be performed. Instruct Sharon how to keep a record of level of fatigue and activities performed. Help Sharon develop a plan to balance activity with level of fatigue.

   Altered body image: Allow Sharon time to express feelings of altered body image; reassure Sharon these feelings are common among SLE clients; encourage Sharon to join a support group for SLE clients where she can discuss this problem with others.

6. What teaching would be done for Sharon's home care?

   Sharon should be taught to maintain a safe environment, schedule planned rest periods, and encourage children to participate in taking care of the home.

7. Identify resources available to help Sharon cope with this chronic condition.

   Lupus Foundation of America, Inc. and the Arthritis Foundation and their local chapters.

ANSWERS TO REVIEW QUESTIONS

1. Ms. Caldwell has just been diagnosed with syphilis and has an order for 1,000,000 units of penicillin I.M. She has no history of allergies to medications. She has never had penicillin. When giving her the injection in the right upper outer quadrant of her buttocks, you note a tattoo. Several minutes after receiving the injection, she tells you she feels anxious and weak. You note she is diaphoretic, scratching her forearm, and is breathing faster than normal. Based upon this assessment data, you would conclude:

   d. these are early signs of an anaphylactic reaction.

2. Which of the following is a potentially life-threatening transfusion reaction?

   a. acute hemolytic reaction

3. Organ transplant clients, living at home and taking immunosuppressive medications, should be encouraged to:

   b. notify their physician if side effects to their medications develop.

4. Sensitivity to sunlight, a butterfly rash and renal failure are symptoms of which of the following conditions?

   d. systemic lupus erythematosus

5. Rheumatoid arthritis is:

   a. an autoimmune disease characterized by abnormal IgG antibodies.

6. Increased muscle weakness, difficulty chewing or swallowing, and shortness of breath in clients with myasthenia gravis are signs of:

   c. both cholinergic crisis and myasthenic crisis.

7. A side effect of corticosteroid medications is:

   d. increased susceptibility to infection.

8. Surgical removal of the thymus gland is useful in controlling symptoms of which of the following conditions?

   b. myasthenia gravis

CHAPTER 25
HIV Disorders

SUGGESTED RESPONSES TO THE CASE STUDY

Jim Hayes, a thirty-seven-year-old male, suspects that he is HIV positive. He enters the medical unit with chronic symptoms such as fever, night sweats, diarrhea, weight loss, shortness of breath, and a nonproductive cough. On the initial assessment he is alert and oriented, color is pale, temperature 100.6°F, pulse 92, respirations 36, and blood pressure 140/70. He has generalized lymphadenopathy. Height 5' 11" and his weight is 125 pounds. Jim states that he is not currently taking any medications although he is "familiar" with the drug AZT.

1. List symptoms/clinical manifestations, other than Mr. Hayes', that a client may experience when HIV positive.
Other symptoms/clinical manifestations a client may experience are: candidiasis, cervical dysplasia, herpes zoster, listeriosis, peripheral neuropathy, loss of appetite, and pain.

2. List two reasons AZT (Retrovir) may be initiated for Mr. Hayes.
Reasons Mr. Hayes may begin taking AZT are: to prevent replication of HIV as prophylactic treatment against opportunistic infections.

3. List two diagnostic tests that will confirm the diagnosis of HIV positive.
Two diagnostic tests that will confirm the diagnosis of HIV positive are: Western blot and polymerase chain reaction (PCR).

4. List subjective and objective data the nurse would want to obtain about Mr. Hayes.
Subjective data: Has he ever had unprotected sexual intercourse or multiple sex partners, traded sex for money or drugs, injected drugs or shared needles. Sexual history.
Objective data: Look for "tracks" on his arms from injecting drugs. Review results of ELISA and/or Western blot tests.

5. Write three individual nursing diagnoses and goals for Mr. Hayes.
Nursing Diagnosis 1: **Breathing pattern, ineffective, related to shortness of breath.**
Goal: **Mr. Hayes will pace activities to minimize shortness of breath.**
Nursing Diagnosis 2: **Fluid volume deficit, related to diarrhea, night sweats, and fever.**
Goal: **Mr. Hayes will have normal skin turgor. Mr. Hayes will have decreased frequency and amount of stools.**
Nursing Diagnosis 3: **Nutrition, altered, less than body requirements, related to diarrhea.**
Goal: **Mr. Hayes will maintain current weight.**

6. List pertinent nursing actions the nurse would do in caring for Mr. Hayes related to:
hydration
fatigue
nutrition
oxygenation
medications
Pertinent nursing actions the nurse would take in caring for Mr. Hayes related to
Hydration—Encourage him to drink liquids between meals
Monitor I&O
Monitor laboratory reports for electrolyte levels.
Fatigue—Alternate activities with rest periods.
Plan care to allow rest periods.
Nutrition—Provide oral hygiene before and after meals.
Have prescribed diet presented to Mr. Hayes as small, frequent meals.
Offer foods that Mr. Hayes likes.
Have foods at room temperature.

Offer nutritional supplements between meals.
Administer prescribed vitamin and mineral supplements.
Oxygenation—Reposition Mr. Hayes at least every two hours.
Administer oxygen as ordered.
Encourage the use of an incentive spirometer.
Medications—Explain expected action and possible side effects of each medication. Administer medications as ordered. Encourage Mr. Hayes to continue taking medications as prescribed.

7. List resources that could assist Mr. Hayes with his diagnosis.
Centers for Disease Control and Prevention
Local Health Department
Local AIDS organizations
American Foundation for AIDS Research
American Red Cross
National Association of People with AIDS
National AIDS/HIV Hotline

8. List teaching Mr. Hayes will need before leaving the medical unit.
Teaching Mr. Hayes will need includes: medications he is taking, nutrition, activity/rest, maintaining fluid balance, identifying symptoms of possible opportunistic infections, need for protected sex, keeping appointments with health care providers.

ANSWERS TO THE REVIEW QUESTIONS

1. Which of the following statements show that the client understands a diagnosis of HIV positive?
c. "Because I am HIV positive I have the virus that causes AIDS."

2. The drug of choice for treating *Pneumocystis carinii* pneumonia (PCP) is:
a. co-trimoxazole (Septra).

3. The nurse is caring for a client who is experiencing diarrhea and weight loss. Which of the following nursing interventions is appropriate for him?
c. offer small, frequent meals

4. The nurse is caring for a client who asks when AZT (Retrovir) is normally started. Which of the following would be the nurse's correct response?
b. when CD4 level reaches 500/mm³

5. The nurse is discussing transmission of HIV with a client. Which of the following statements indicates that the client needs more education?
d. "I should not hug or kiss anyone."

6. The only opportunistic infection that is found when the CD4 cell count is normal is:
b. Kaposi's sarcoma.

CHAPTER 26

Musculoskeletal Disorders

SUGGESTED RESPONSES TO THE CASE STUDY

George Ellis, a forty-year-old truck driver, was getting ready to help unload his cargo. He was climbing into the truck when he lost his balance and fell to the ground twisting his left leg. He stated he was in severe pain and was unable to stand. His coworkers called the emergency ambulance service to transport him to the hospital. Upon arrival in the emergency room, the nurse immediately took Mr. Ellis's vital signs. His vital signs were temperature

98.6°F, pulse 92, respirations 24, and blood pressure 158/90. The nurse also noted that Mr. Ellis's face was flushed and his left leg was shorter than his right.

1. List five types of fractures.
    compound, greenstick, pathologic, impacted or telescoped, spiral

2. Based on the action of the fall, what type of fracture do you think Mr. Ellis received?
    spiral

3. What diagnostic measures will determine whether or not Mr. Ellis has a fracture of his left leg?
    x-ray, CT Scan

4. What immediate care should have been given to Mr. Ellis?
    Avoid moving the affected leg; let it remain in the same position at the time of Mr. Ellis's fall. Keep Mr. Ellis warm.

3. List four nursing interventions for clients in traction.
    Administer pain medication as prescribed; assess skin over bony prominences for redness; make sure weights hang freely; perform a neurological assessment of body part in traction.

6. What options may be considered for treatment of Mr. Ellis' injury?
    Mr. Ellis's leg may be casted or placed in skeletal traction, depending on the severity of the fracture.

7. List objective and subjective information the nurse would obtain regarding Mr. Ellis's injury.
    Subjective: **Mr. Ellis stated he couldn't stand on his leg, twisted his leg when he fell, was in severe pain.**
    Objective: **Left leg shorter than right leg, flushed skin, rapid pulse and respirations, blood pressure elevated.**

ANSWERS TO THE REVIEW QUESTIONS

1. Upon admission to the hospital the client expresses concerns for his job. This information will become which part of his nursing care plan?
    c. Validating factor.

2. A fracture caused by forceful twisting is known as what kind of a fracture?
    b. Spiral.

3. The primary goal in the treatment of a fracture is to:
    d. prevent further injury to the fractured limb.

4. A closed reduction of a fracture:
    b. is completed by manual manipulation.

5. Poor body positioning and alignment of an immobilized client may result in deformities. One of the deformities that may develop is:
    c. contracture.

6. One of the first symptoms a client with arthritis may complain of is:
    b. joint stiffness, especially on arising.

7. Areas of the body most often affected by arthritis are:
    a. knees, hips, fingers.

8. Braces, casts, or splints may be applied to joints that are painful or in spasm. This is done to prevent:
    a. deformities.

9. Traction is frequently used to treat clients with a musculoskeletal problem. One of the primary reasons for traction is to:
    b. maintain a corrected position.

10. Osteomyelitis:
    b. is a bacterial infection of the bone.

CHAPTER 27
Nervous System Disorders

SUGGESTED RESPONSES TO THE CASE STUDY

Mr. George Mason, a seventy-six-year-old retired farmer, was admitted to the emergency room with a left-sided hemiplegia, difficulty swallowing, and inability to speak. He was awake and watching the staff upon admission. He moved his right arm to indicate that Mrs. Mason was his wife, but was unable to speak or form sounds. Mr. Mason stated that he was working in the garden picking tomatoes and cucumbers when he fell to the ground thirty minutes before admission. The emergency room nurse administered oxygen per nasal cannula at 2 liters per minute and obtained vital signs. His blood pressure was 182/98, pulse was 88, respirations were 20, and temperature was 100.5°F. The emergency room physician ordered a MRI scan of the head STAT, a complete blood count, and prothrombin time. The MRI indicated that Mr. Mason experienced a cerebrovascular accident caused by a bleeding into the brain.

1. List clinical manifestations other than the ones Mr. Mason experienced that can occur when having a cerebrovascular accident.
   Clinical manifestations that can occur with a CVA other than the hemiplegia, dysphagia, and aphasia that Mr. Mason experienced are: hemiparesis, dysarthria, emotional lability, loss of emotional control, inability to control behavior, inability to process multiple pieces of information, agnosia, inability to recognize familiar objects

2. List subjective and objective data a nurse would want to obtain.
   Subjective data: **visual problems, headache, numbness of tingling feelings, ability to think, confusion, overwhelmed feeling.**
   Objective data: **Neurological assessment for: level of consciousness, motor function, sensation, cranial nerve function, swallowing ability, signs and symptoms of increased intracranial pressure, mental status, intellectual status, functional ability to perform activities of daily living, knowledge status of disease process, spatial perceptual deficits, and also vital signs.**

3. Identify three individualized nursing diagnoses and goals for Mr. Mason.
   Nursing Diagnosis 1: **Communication, impaired verbal, related to neuromuscular impairment.**
   Goal: **Mr. Mason will communicate needs for toileting, changing position, and social interaction to the nursing staff by using a communication board.**
   Nursing Diagnosis 2: **Self-care deficit, related to inability to use left arm.**
   Goal: **Mr. Mason will have all self-care needs met.**
   Nursing Diagnosis 3: **Unilateral neglect, left, related to spatial-perceptual deficit secondary to neuromuscular impairment.**
   Goal: **Mr. Mason will not incur injury to the left side of his body.**

4. Mr. Mason is transferred to a general medical unit for three days, then is transferred to a rehabilitation center for intensive therapy. What pertinent nursing actions should a nurse perform in caring for Mr. Mason in the acute setting and the rehabilitation setting related to (see page 72):
   Mobility   Elimination
   Skin Integrity   Comfort/Rest
   Safety

5. List teaching that Mr. Mason will need before discharge from the rehabilitation facility.
   Mobility; assistive devices; skin care; disease process; bowel elimination; bladder elimination; safety management; nutritional/dysphagia management; medications—dosage, frequency, actions, side effects; compensation for unilateral neglect; activities of daily living

Acute Care	Rehabilitation
MOBILITY Turn Mr. Mason every 1–2 hours. Perform range of motion every 2–4 hours to prevent contractures. Plexipulse boots to prevent thrombophlebitis and deep vein thrombosis.	Collaborate with physical therapy and occupational therapy in increasing functional ability. Maintain splint protocol of applying and removing as scheduled by therapies. Perform range of motion to all joints at least four times per day. Teach Mr. Mason to perform range of motion as possible. Teach Mr. Mason to move his affected arm, hands, fingers, and legs using his unaffected limbs. Assess for signs and symptoms of complications of immobility such as pressure areas, pneumonia, and deep vein thrombosis. Use a consistent approach when moving and transferring Mr. Mason in order to promote his education and increase his independence.
SAFETY Maintain seizure precautions. Protect him from falls. Teach Mr. Mason to call for assistance to transfer. Place call light within his reach. Cue Mr. Mason to attend to his left side, to watch where he is walking, and to keep his left arm away from wheels of the wheelchair. Maintain an uncluttered environment with necessary supplies within his reach. Observe Mr. Mason for swallowing difficulties, aspiration, or signs and symptoms of pneumonia.	Stimulate Mr. Mason's awareness of the neglected side by having him perform tasks using the neglected side, touching the neglected side, or bring the neglected side into his line of vision to reacquaint him with his body. Cue Mr. Mason to watch the neglected side and the environment on that side to prevent injury from walking into a wall or injuring his hand in the wheels of the wheelchair. Assess for visual problems, and teach Mr. Mason to compensate for loss of vision.
ELIMINATION Assess elimination patterns for continence and incontinence. Monitor fluid balance. Monitor for constipation related to decreased mobility and change in routine.	Implement a bowel and bladder retraining program. Toilet Mr. Mason every two hours and monitor his ability to maintain continence. Administer suppositories or laxatives to establish a bowel elimination pattern. Provide plenty of bulk and fluids to promote bowel elimination. Catheterize intermittently for neurogenic bladder.
SKIN INTEGRITY Assess condition of skin every 4 hours; turn every 1–2 hours; massage pressure points with lotion; when up in chair change position frequently to prevent pressure areas.	Continue to assess skin condition. Observe for shearing of skin from moving and transferring. Assess skin under splints. Teach Mr. Mason to observe condition of skin.
COMFORT/REST Maintain a quiet environment to decrease stimuli. Provide comfort measures such as back rubs and warm blankets. Keep Mr. Mason informed of what is happening by speaking slowly and concisely to allow him to process the information. Allow family/significant others to spend time with him. Turn and position frequently.	Establish a routine that provides for rest periods between activities to increase activity tolerance. Gradually increase length of therapies. Focus on the coping abilities of Mr. Mason and his family. Provide emotional support to Mr. Mason and family. Assess for apathy, emotional lability, and depression.

6.   List at least three client outcomes for Mr. Mason.

    (1) Mr. Mason performs self care with minimal assistance.

    (2) Mr. Mason communicates daily needs through verbal communication and the use of a sign board.

    (3) Mr. Mason integrates the left side of his body into his body image.

    (4) Mr. Mason safely transfers from bed to wheelchair and wheelchair to toilet and back with standby assist of one person.

    (5) Mr. Mason maintains continence of bowel and bladder.

ANSWERS TO THE REVIEW QUESTIONS

1. The most important indicator of neurological status is:
   a. level of consciousness.
2. Cranial nerves III, IV, and VI all have functions affecting:
   c. eye movement.
3. Assessment of intellectual function requires that the nurse:
   a. have knowledge of the client's prior ability to function.
4. Contusion of the brain is a (an):
   d. bruising of the brain.
5. Benign brain tumors can be:
   d. the cause of increased intracranial pressure.
6. Miss Webster, a 24-year-old client with Guillain-Barre Syndrome can be told which of the following:
   b. the disease is an acute inflammatory process with most clients regaining complete function.

CHAPTER 28

Sensory Disorders

SUGGESTED RESPONSES TO THE CASE STUDY

Katie Rollins is a thirty-four-year-old nurse who was diagnosed with a right ear hearing impairment during a routine physical exam. She admitted to her doctor that she noticed she would only use her left ear to talk on the phone and that she had particular difficulty hearing her family or friends in a crowded restaurant or other public settings. She also noted that her husband asked her why she played the TV so loud, yet if he turned it down to his normal hearing level, she could not hear it clearly. Her physician ordered an audiogram which showed a conductive hearing loss of 40 percent secondary to otosclerosis. Hearing in her left ear was normal.

Katie's doctor gave her three medical treatment options.

1. Do nothing and monitor her hearing impairment by audiogram every six months. If it were to worsen, other options would be considered.
2. Be fitted with a hearing aid.
3. Have a surgical procedure to correct the hearing loss.

Katie agreed to have surgery. She thought she would be too self-conscious to wear a hearing aid, after all she was only thirty-four, but she simply could not ignore the problem by doing nothing. Katie was scheduled for same-day surgery.

1. What diagnostic tests were done on the initial exam to diagnose a conductive hearing loss? List other diagnostic tests that may have been ordered for Katie.
   Weber test and Rinne test. Other tests that may have been ordered include otoscopic exam, audiometric testing, speech audiometry, and CT scan or MRI.
2. How is a conductive hearing loss differentiated from a sensorineural hearing loss?
   During the tuning fork tests, if the sound is louder when the tines are placed beside the ear, then hearing is normal or the hearing loss is sensorineural. If the sound is louder when conducted through bone, then the hearing loss is conductive.

3. What does an audiogram tell you? What special things should Katie know before she has the audiogram?
The audiogram can detect both bone and air conduction and determine the degree of hearing loss. She will be in a soundproof booth during the audiometric testing.

4. Describe the surgical procedure that will most likely be used to correct the conductive hearing loss.
The surgical procedure most likely to be used is a stapedectomy. A surgical incision is made in the posterior portion of the ear canal, the stapes is removed and a prosthesis is placed.

5. What will you teach Katie prior to her surgery about the procedure and expected postoperative course?
Preoperative teaching should include a description of the surgical procedure and expected results. Katie will be NPO and possibly stay overnight. Teaching should also include expected pain control, activity restrictions, and the need to call for assistance if ambulating. In addition, Katie should expect vertigo and be instructed that medication is available to lessen the effects of vertigo. If Katie will be discharged on antibiotics, medication teaching should include precautions to complete the dose. The follow-up appointment and need to avoid water in or around the operative ear is necessary.

6. List four individualized nursing diagnoses and expected outcomes for Katie and nursing interventions for each diagnosis.
(1) Anxiety related to a decrease or loss of hearing.
Nursing interventions:
Encourage Katie to ask questions about procedure and anticipated outcome. Provide honest and realistic feedback.
(2) Knowledge deficit related to preoperative preparations and postoperative care.
Nursing interventions:
Provide written and verbal information on the procedure, risks, and expected results and what not to do postoperatively. Answer questions knowledgeably and in terms the client understands. Clarify NPO status. Suggest bringing an overnight bag in case it is needed. Instruct client to wear hair up to avoid betadine prep solution from getting into hair. Discuss postop care related to pain control, antiemetic, antibiotics, bed rest, and activity restrictions such as avoiding sudden movements, blowing nose, and sneezing.
(3) Injury, high risk for, related to vertigo.
Nursing interventions:
Keep side rails up. Instruct the client to move or turn slowly. Reiterate need to call for assistance when ambulating. Keep call bell within reach. Administer medications for vertigo prior to worsening of symptoms. Keep room well lit when ambulating.
(4) Injury, high risk for, related to displacement of prosthesis.
Nursing interventions:
Maintain bed rest for 24–48 hours. Remind client to avoid sudden movement, sneezing, or nose blowing. Monitor vital signs q4h. Be particularly attentive to temperature for evidence of infection, excessive clear or bloody drainage, and pain not controlled with prescribed analgesics. Administer analgesics and/or sedatives to reduce discomfort and promote rest.
(5) Knowledge deficit related to surgical aftercare.
Nursing interventions:
Teach client how and when to perform dressing change. Have client demonstrate the procedure. Instruct client to avoid pressure changes (such as flying in an unpressurized aircraft) and avoid heavy lifting (> 60 lbs.) for one month. Avoid nose blowing for 10 days. If sneezing occurs, keep mouth open. Keep water out of the ear and keep the ear exposed to air as much as possible for one month. Expect some drainage which is initially red, then pink, and then brownish as the dissolvable pack works its way out of the ear. Report any greenish, yellowish, or foul-smelling drainage. Take all antibiotics as prescribed and complete full course of treatment. You should experience very little pain or discomfort. Take prescribed analgesics and notify doctor for prolonged or intense pain. Hearing may be decreased for 3–4 weeks after surgery until gelfoam packing dissolves. Audiometric testing will be conducted one month after surgery. The first appointment is in one month. You may be seen sooner if you experience any uncontrolled pain or malodorous, greenish discharge from your ear. Call your doctor immediately.

7. How might Katie's pain be controlled?
Pain control can be achieved with oral, intramuscular, or suppository analgesics.

8. Describe the expected discharge instructions that Katie must know related to diet, medications, activity restrictions, and follow-up care.

When she goes home there are no dietary restrictions. However, if she has to sneeze, she should keep her mouth open so pressure does not increase in her eustachian tube. Avoid heavy lifting for one month. Avoid blowing nose for 10 days. Keep water out of ear and keep ear open to air for one month. Report any greenish, yellowish, or foul-smelling drainage to the physician. Take all of the antibiotics prescribed. Keep doctor's appointment in one month.

ANSWERS TO REVIEW QUESTIONS

1. The three bones of the middle ear are:
   d. malleus, incus, stapes.
2. In a conductive hearing loss:
   c. sound waves are not transmitted through the ear canal to inner ear fluid.
3. A possible nursing diagnosis for a client with Meniere's disease is:
   c. communication, impaired, verbal, related to tinnitus.
4. Persons with hearing impairment or loss may benefit from:
   d. cupping the ear and turning the head toward the person speaking to them.
5. Chemical burns of the eye are treated with:
   c. flushing of the lids, conjunctiva, and cornea with water.
6. Postoperatively, the client who has cataract surgery should be placed:
   d. supine with a small pillow under the head.
7. Increased ocular pressure is indicated by a reading of:
   d. 23 to 30 mmHg.
8. A clinical symptom of a detached retina is:
   c. momentary flashes of light.
9. Macular degeneration is characterized by:
   c. loss of central vision.

CHAPTER 29

Endocrine Disorders

SUGGESTED RESPONSES TO THE CASE STUDY

Mary Jane Trudell, forty-three years of age, was diagnosed with Addison's disease when she was thirty-four years old and placed on long-term steroid therapy. Due to sudden financial problems, she was unable to refill her prescription for steroids. She came to the emergency room with a rapid onset of fatigue, muscle weakness, lightheadedness upon rising, weight loss, and a craving for salty foods. She is anxious, irritable, and slightly confused. She is diagnosed as being in Addisonian crisis and admitted to the hospital. Her orders include: vital signs q4h, IV of D-5-RL @ 125 cc/hr continuous, Solu-Cortef 100 mg IVP now, then IVPB q8h, regular diet, bed rest with bathroom privileges.

1. Discuss the difference in clinical manifestations between Addison's disease and adrenal crisis.
   The clinical manifestations are basically the same; however, the onset of the clinical manifestations is much quicker in adrenal crisis.

2. Discuss vital signs the nurse should expect to find when assessing Ms. Trudell.
   Ms. Trudell may experience hypotension with a weak irregular pulse. As treatment continues, the blood pressure and pulse should return to normal limits.

3. List three nursing diagnoses and goals for Ms. Trudell.
   Nursing Diagnosis 1: **fluid volume deficit related to decreased sodium levels, as evidenced by vomiting, diarrhea, and increased renal losses.**
   Goal: **Ms. Trudell's sodium level will return to normal and remain stable.**
   Nursing Diagnosis 2: **Infection, high risk for, related to suppressed inflammatory response.**
   Goal: **Ms. Trudell will remain free of infection.**
   Nursing Diagnosis 3: **Knowledge deficit, related to inadequate understanding of decreased adrenal function and steroid therapy as evidenced by not having steroid prescription filled.**
   Goal: **Ms. Trudell will verbalize cause and symptoms of decreased adrenal function and withdrawal symptoms of steroid therapy.**
   Nursing Diagnosis 4: **Tissue perfusion, altered, related to fluid loss as evidenced by lightheadedness.**
   Goal: **Ms. Trudell will not experience symptoms of altered tissue perfusion such as lightheadedness.**
   Nursing Diagnosis 4: **Injury, high risk for, related to confusion or impaired judgment.**
   Goal: **Ms. Trudell will not suffer injury during hospitalization.**

4. List teaching that Ms. Trudell will need concerning long-term steroid use.
   Steroids need to be taken for a lifetime. Take steroids with foods or antacids. Maintain a diet high in protein and potassium and low in sodium. Take in divided doses. Steroids can interfere with oral contraceptive effectiveness. Steroids can mask severe infections. Wounds will heal slower. Contact a physician before taking over-the-counter medications. Dosage should be tapered. Do not discontinue abruptly. Wear a medic alert bracelet.

5. List three successful outcomes for Ms. Trudell.
   (1) **Ms. Trudell will verbalize understanding of her disease process and continued need to be monitored by a physician.**
   (2) **Ms. Trudell will verbalize understanding of her medication regimen and when she should seek medical help.**
   (3) **Ms. Trudell will verbalize understanding of stress reduction and relaxation techniques.**

ANSWERS TO THE REVIEW QUESTIONS

1. Explanations prior to diagnostic tests for an endocrine disorder are most important to
   d. reduce stress that can interfere with test results.
2. Which of the following nursing diagnoses would be most appropriate for the client with diabetes insipidus?
   c. Fluid volume deficit related to polyuria
3. Meticulous skin care is especially important for the client with hyperthyroidism because of:
   a. diaphoresis from heat intolerance.
4. The nurse would assess for which of the following clinical manifestations in the client with hypothyroidism?
   c. unexplained weight gain, energy loss, and cold intolerance
5. The client with hyperparathyroidism should have extremities handled gently because:
   a. decreased calcium bone deposits can lead to pathologic fractures.
6. Which of the following assessments would the nurse expect to observe in the client with pheochromocytoma?
   d. systolic pressure up to 300 mmHg

CHAPTER 30

Diabetes Mellitus

SUGGESTED RESPONSES TO THE CASE STUDY

Mr. Carnes, a forty-four-year-old African American male, is admitted to the medical unit from his physician's office. He reports that he has lost 18 pounds over the last month and has been very tired. He also reports symptoms of thirst, frequent urination, and blurred vision. His vital signs are: BP 166/92, P 88, R 16, T 99.2°F. Physical assessment reveals hot, dry, flushed skin. Laboratory exams reveal a blood glucose 490 mg/dL and urine negative for ketones. Mr. Carnes is a truck driver and leads a fairly sedentary lifestyle. History reveals that he is usually 30 to 35 pounds overweight, but has otherwise been in good health. He reports that his mother died from diabetes and renal failure, and an older brother was diagnosed as having NIDDM three years ago.

1. List physical symptoms that Mr. Carnes is experiencing which are suggestive of diabetes.
   Symptoms include: weight loss, fatigue, thirst, polyuria, blurred vision, and hot, dry, flushed skin.

2. Based on history and laboratory values, would you expect Mr. Carnes to be diagnosed with IDDM or NIDDM?
   NIDDM (characterized by adult-onset, presence of obesity, urine negative for ketones)

3. Which nursing diagnoses would you identify as priority for Mr. Carnes right now? List two.
   Possible diagnoses could include:
   Fluid volume deficit, related to polyuria and dehydration.
   Knowledge deficit, disease and treatment, self-care skills.
   Nutrition, altered, less than body requirements, related to disease process

4. Mr. Carnes is treated with IV fluids and insulin sliding scale until his blood glucose is stabilized. Describe what an insulin sliding scale is, and when it is used.
   Insulin sliding scale is used to stabilize serum glucose during times of illness, surgery, or stress. Regular insulin is administered every 4 hours based on blood glucose level (usually measured by SMBG).

5. A 2,000 calorie ADA diet is ordered for Mr. Carnes. Mr. Carnes does not care to eat the apple that came on his breakfast tray and asks if he can exchange it for another serving of scrambled eggs. How would you respond to Mr. Carnes?
   Eggs belong to the meat (protein) group and should not be substituted for a fruit. Another fruit exchange would be an appropriate substitute, e.g., ½ banana or 1 apple.

6. Mr. Carnes is being discharged and will continue to attend diabetic education classes at a local diabetic treatment center. Assuming Mr. Carnes is to continue on a diabetic diet and will be receiving mixed insulin injections, list the pertinent information Mr. Carnes will need to know about his disease and therapies related to:

   - Diabetes and symptoms of hyperglycemia
   - Role of exercise
   - Effects of diet
   - Self-monitoring blood glucose
   - Insulin injections/technique
   - Symptoms of hypoglycemia
   - Sick day care
   - Long-term complications

   Diabetes and symptoms of hyperglycemia:
   In addition to usual symptoms of polyuria, polydipsia, and polyphagia, often experience fatigue, visual changes, paresthesias, and recurrent infections.

Role of exercise: Exercise decreases blood glucose by increasing the uptake of glucose by body muscles and improving insulin usage. Exercise also increases circulation, improves cardiovascular status, decreases stress, and assists with weight loss. Regular daily exercise is better than sporadic exercise. Avoid exercising when blood glucose is too high or too low.

Effects of diet: Should eat at consistent time synchronized with the action of the insulin. Distribute calories over 24 hours with regular meals and snacks.

Self-monitoring blood glucose: Assure that Mr. Carnes understands the use of the specific home glucose monitoring equipment he is to use.

Insulin injections/technique: How to store the insulin. How to draw up the regular insulin first, then the longer-acting insulin. Insulin is given in subcutaneous fat; the abdomen gives the most predictable absorption. Use syringe and needle only once.

Symptoms of hypoglycemia: Can occur anytime, but most generally before meals or at peak insulin action. Generally are sudden and unexpected. Include diaphoresis, pallor, palpitations, hunger, tremors, paresthesias, and anxiety. May progress to slurred speech, confusion, behavior changes, disorientation, seizures, or loss of consciousness.

Sick day care: Have a plan for illness. Continue to take insulin. Monitor blood glucose 4–6 times a day and check urine for ketones. Blood glucose over 300 gm/dL should be reported to the physician. If he cannot eat planned meals should have carbohydrates as soft foods and liquids. Extreme nausea, vomiting, or diarrhea should be reported to the physician.

Long-term complications: More prone to infections, especially foot infections, cellulitis, urinary tract infections, and yeast infections.

   Neuropathy—causes paresthesias and burning sensations, primarily in the lower extremities. There is decreased sensations of pain and temperature. More prone to constipation, diarrhea, urine retention, and impotence (male).

   Nephropathy—develops slowly. Twenty to 40 percent chance of developing renal disease and renal failure.

   Retinopathy—changes in small vessels of retina leads to blindness. Develop cataracts at earlier age.

   Vascular changes—atherosclerotic changes appear at an earlier age and progress more rapidly. Hypertension twice as common as in non-diabetic. Peripheral vascular disease more common with hypertension.

ANSWERS TO THE REVIEW QUESTIONS

1. Mrs. Gavin tells the nurse that she is surprised that she developed diabetes at 40 years of age. The nurse knows that the development of diabetes in middle-aged people is most directly the result of:
   c. obesity.
2. Glycosylated HgA is:
   a. a blood test that shows the pattern of blood glucose levels over several months.
3. When teaching the diabetic client about mixing short- and longer-acting (NPH) insulin in the same syringe, the nurse should teach that:
   a. regular insulin should be drawn up first.
4. Which of the following principles is used when planning for a diabetic who is to undergo surgery?
   c. Sliding scale insulin is used to regulate glucose levels during the operative period.
5. Mr. Schultz and the nurse collaborate to establish a meal plan for his 1,800 calorie ADA diet. The principle used in the exchange system are based on the fact that Mr. Schultz:
   b. may substitute any food in the correct amount for another on the same exchange list.
6. JoAnne is a twenty-one-year-old college student who has been diagnosed with IDDM for seven years. In reviewing principles of insulin administration with JoAnne, the nurse knows that she understands the relationship of her food intake and action of regular insulin when she tells the nurse she eats:
   a. within 30 minutes after her insulin injection.
7. Ms. Perez, who has IDDM, complains of weakness and shakiness. She is pale, diaphoretic, and her pulse rate is increased. The nurse should recognize these symptoms as indications of:
   b. hypoglycemia.

8. Mrs. Lally, age twenty-four, is a newly diagnosed insulin-dependent diabetic. If Mrs. Lally's husband comes home and finds her unconscious, what is the first thing he should do?

    a. place some easily absorbed glucose under her tongue (e.g., monogel) or give glucagon SC or IM.

9. You have been teaching Mr. Morales to give himself insulin injections. Which of the following statements indicates that he understands what you've taught him?

    b. "I'll clean the injection site carefully before administering."

10. To which one of the following diseases is the diabetic most predisposed?

    c. Atherosclerosis

CHAPTER 31
Female Reproductive Disorders

SUGGESTED RESPONSES TO THE CASE STUDY

Mrs. Mary Keiver, a forty-year-old, African American school teacher, nullipara, was seen by her physician because of heavy menstrual bleeding. She stated that she had been saturating a sanitary pad every thirty minutes since early that same morning. She reported that her menstrual periods had been getting heavier for the past six months and were accompanied by severe cramping. She also noted that after her period she felt "physically drained." Other symptoms that Mary had observed included an increasing sense of heaviness in her pelvis and her skirts and slacks were too tight around the abdomen, even though her weight had not changed significantly. When Mary was examined by the physician, it was noted that her uterus was enlarged approximately equal to twelve weeks gestational size and it felt irregular in shape. Mary's skin was pale and cool to touch. Her mucous membranes and conjunctival sacs were pale pink. Her blood pressure was 100/60, pulse 90, temperature 98.8°F. The results of an H & H were as follows: Hgb = 7.0 mg/dL and HCT = 26. An ultrasound confirmed the findings of the pelvic exam for the presence of multiple uterine fibroids. The bleeding did not subside, and Mary was admitted for an outpatient dilatation and curettage (D&C) with a diagnosis of menorrhagia secondary to uterine leiomyoma.

1. List the clinical signs and symptoms manifested by this client that suggest that the heavy bleeding may be related to uterine fibroids.

    Clinical signs and symptoms that suggest the heavy bleeding may be related to uterine fibroids are:
        nulliparous
        African American
        excessively heavy menstrual flow
        abdominal enlargement
        increasing sense of heaviness in pelvis

2. List two reasons why a hemoglobin and hematocrit were ordered.

    Reasons for ordering a hemoglobin and hematocrit are: hemoglobin identifies the oxygen-carrying capability of the RBCs, and hematocrit identifies the percentage of the blood that is RBCs. Together they show how well body tissues may be oxygenated.

3. Describe what other diagnostic tests were ordered and why.

    The other diagnostic test ordered was an ultrasound. It would identify the presence of fibroids.

4. List the subjective and objective data the nurse should obtain during the assessment.

    Subjective data: **Menstrual history, obstetrical history, knowledge and feelings about the excessive bleeding, dysmenorrhea, menorrhagia, increasing pelvic pressure, abdominal enlargement but no weight gain, pelvic pain.**

Objective data: Number of vaginal pads saturated per hour, presence of clots, low hemoglobin and hematocrit levels, pale skin, pulse increased, irregularities palpated on uterus, and ultrasound showing fibroids.

5. Write three individualized nursing diagnoses and goals for Mrs. Keiver.
    Nursing Diagnosis 1: **Fluid volume deficit, high risk for, related to excessive blood loss.**
    Goal: **Mrs. Keiver will maintain fluid balance.**
    Nursing Diagnosis 2: **Anxiety, related to active blood loss, hospitalization, and pending surgery.**
    Goal: **Mrs. Keiver will discuss fears and concerns with health care givers.**
    Nursing Diagnosis 3: **Pain, related to cramping during menses, and pressure on pelvic structures caused by growing fibroids.**
    Goal: **Mrs. Keiver will verbalize having less discomfort and pelvic pressure.**

6. Describe pertinent nursing actions/interventions to be taken in caring for this client prior to and following the D&C related to:

    • Bleeding
    • Cardiac output
    • Comfort/rest
    • Activity
    • Medications
    • Teaching

    Nursing actions to be taken for Mrs. Keiver prior to and following the D&C related to:
    Bleeding—Prior to D&C
        check vaginal pad saturation frequently
        check vital signs
    Following D&C
        check vaginal pad for bleeding
        check vital signs
    Cardiac Output—Prior to and following D&C
        check pulse and blood pressure
    Comfort/rest—Prior to D&C
        administer ordered pain medication
        give back rub
        change vaginal pad frequently
    Following D&C
        assist to change position
        administer ordered pain medication
    Activity—Prior to D&C
        bed rest
    Following D&C
        ambulate as ordered
    Medications—Prior to and following D&C
        ask if Mrs. Keiver has any allergies
        explain what each medication is given for and the expected result
    Teaching—Prior to D&C
        provide Mrs. Keiver with the information about what will be happening until the D&C is performed and what to expect postoperatively
    Following D&C
        reinforce teaching about postoperative period

7. List a minimum of three specific topics the nurse should discuss when talking to this client regarding her condition.
    Topics to discuss with Mrs. Keiver are: plans regarding having a family, amount of standing required in her job, the tightness of her clothes around her abdomen

8. Discuss discharge instructions or teaching necessary for this client.
    Discharge instructions or teaching:

inform physician the next time she has a heavy period, no heavy lifting until seen again by physician, adequate fluid intake, diet high in iron, taking prescribed medications as ordered

9. List a minimum of three successful outcomes for this client.
    Successful outcomes:
    Fluid balance is maintained. Hemoglobin and hematocrit levels increase to normal range. Menstrual flow is not excessive.

10. Discuss how the nurse might evaluate the effectiveness of treatment and care for this client.
    Evaluate the effectiveness of treatment and care:
    Goals related to nursing diagnoses are met. Successful outcomes are fulfilled.

ANSWERS TO THE REVIEW QUESTIONS

1. The best method of screening for cervical cancer is:
    c. Pap smear.
2. The client should perform BSE (breast self-examination):
    b. just after the menstrual period.
3. The "silent killer" of many women is:
    d. ovarian cancer.
4. If the client complains of heavy bleeding between her normal menstrual cycles it is called:
    c. metorrhagia.
5. Bowel and bladder complications that may follow pelvic radiation therapy for uterine cancer are often caused by:
    c. damage to the tissue from radiation effects.
6. The most common cancer of the female reproductive system is:
    a. breast.
7. An example of an antiestrogenic drug used in the treatment of female reproductive cancers, especially in breast cancer, is:
    a. Megace.
8. The primary microorganism associated with the occurrence of toxic shock syndrome is:
    c. *Staphylococcus aureus.*
9. An example of a barrier method of contraception is:
    a. condom.
10. A dietary element frequently associated with fibrocystic breast disease is:
    d. caffeine.
11. Bright red vaginal bleeding, cramping, and cervical dilation during the first trimester of pregnancy are symptoms of which type of abortion?
    d. inevitable
12. Which of the following are characteristic signs of a trichomonas vaginitis?
    c. creamy, thin, vaginal discharge with a musty/fishy odor
13. The drug of choice to treat PID (pelvic inflammatory disease) is:
    b. doxycycline.
14. What degree of prolapse is described when the cervix and the uterus extend out of the body, past the vaginal opening?
    c. third degree

CHAPTER 32

Male Reproductive Disorders

SUGGESTED RESPONSES TO THE CASE STUDY

Mr. Able is a seventy-year-old male with a diagnosis of benign prostatic hypertrophy. Prior to his hospital admission for a TURP he has been in good health. He returned from surgery three hours ago with a three-way Foley catheter and continuous bladder irrigation. His vital signs one hour ago were as follows: temperature 98.9°F, apical pulse 68, blood pressure 130/84, and respirations 18. When the nurse enters his room to take another set of vitals, Mr. Able is restless, moaning, has cool, moist skin, and his catheter is not draining properly. His pulse is now 120 and blood pressure is 88/50. The nurse calls the physician to report the change in Mr. Able's condition. The physician orders a STAT hematocrit and a bleeding and clotting time. An increase in the IV fluid drip rate is also ordered. The doctor is planning to arrive at the hospital within the next hour.

1. List symptoms/clinical manifestations, other than Mr. Able's, a client may experience following a TURP.
    The client may experience signs and symptoms of hypervolemia, which include hypertension, bradycardia, weakness, and seizures.

2. List reasons why the doctor has ordered the STAT blood work and the IV changes.
    The doctor has ordered blood work to determine if Mr. Able is hemorrhaging and the IV drip rate has been changed to increase his fluid volume and avoid hemorrhagic shock while waiting for the laboratory report.

3. List other diagnostic tests that may have been ordered for Mr. Able.
    CBC, platelets

4. Mentally do a head-to-toe or functional assessment on Mr. Able. List subjective and objective data a nurse would want to obtain.
    pain
    vital signs every 15 minutes
    input and output
    assess urinary drainage for color and presence of clots
    LOC
    skin color and capillary refill

5. Write three individualized nursing diagnoses and goals for Mr. Able.
    Nursing Diagnosis 1: **Fluid volume deficit, high risk for, related to hemorrhage**
    Goal: **The client will not demonstrate signs of hypovolemia.**
    Nursing Diagnosis 2: **Pain, related to tissue trauma and spasms**
    Goal: **The client will verbalize pain relief and be able to rest comfortably.**
    Nursing Diagnosis 3: **Infection, high risk for, related to invasive procedures of the urinary tract**
    Goal: **The client will remain free of infection.**

6. Upon assessing Mr. Able, the doctor decides to inject additional fluid into the balloon that anchors the indwelling catheter and apply increased traction to the catheter. List pertinent nursing actions a nurse would do following these medical interventions:
    medications: **assess vital signs before administering pain medications.**
    comfort/rest: **make sure that urine is draining freely; reposition, milk, or irrigate the catheter tubing as necessary; administer pain medications as ordered.**
    cardiac output: **monitor for excessive bleeding; assess for signs of hypovolemia or hypervolemia; maintain traction on the catheter.**
    intake and output: **monitor urine for excessive bleeding; maintain flow of irrigating fluid; assess bladder for distention.**

activity: **assess vital signs before allowing out of bed and assist with ambulation; encourage activity when vital signs are stable.**

teaching: **explain rationale for physician adding fluid into the catheter balloon and applying increased traction to the catheter, instruct the client not to release or decrease traction on catheter.**

7. List resources within the medical center and the local area that could assist Mr. Able with his postoperative recovery.

    Sex therapist, marriage counseling, support group

8. List teaching that Mr. Able will need before his discharge.

    Provide information about possible affects of prostatectomy; provide information about signs and symptoms of possible complications; provide information about possible sexual dysfunction; teach how to do perineal exercises; instruct to maintain high fluid intake; if discharged with a catheter, teach how to care for it; encourage ambulation but avoid heavy lifting

9. List at least three successful outcomes for Mr. Able.

    1. **Mr. Able had no symptoms of hypovolemia upon discharge.**
    2. **Mr. Able was able to control pain at a 1–3 level with medication. He was not experiencing bladder spasms on discharge.**
    3. **Mr. Able showed no signs of infection when discharged.**

ANSWERS TO THE REVIEW QUESTIONS

1. Which of the following is the most common site of cancer in the male reproductive system?

    d. prostate

2. Which of the following factors predisposes males to penile cancer?

    b. not being circumcised

3. Which of the following self-examinations should a young man be taught to do?

    d. testicular

4. Which of the following complications may occur after a TURP?

    a. water intoxication

5. Which of the following methods may be used for clearing obstructed catheter tubing post-TURP?

    a. milking the tubing

6. Which of the following is a cause of male infertility?

    d. frequent hot tub or sauna usage

7. Which of the following is a cause of impotency?

    c. Peyronie's disease

8. The purpose of post-TURP continuous bladder irrigation is to

    b. reduce clot formation.

9. Which of the following nursing interventions can help alleviate bladder spasms post-TURP?

    c. administering B&O suppositories

10. Which of the following is a method that can be used to assess the client's level of knowledge related to his inflammatory disorder of the reproductive system?

    d. asking the client to describe the symptoms of his disorder.

CHAPTER 33
Sexually Transmitted Diseases

SUGGESTED RESPONSES TO THE CASE STUDY

> *Noelle Landers, a seventeen-year-old student, has come to your clinic seeking treatment. Noelle is complaining of pain and burning on urination, as well as pain during intercourse. She states that she is infrequently sexually active with her seventeen-year-old boyfriend, and is also seeking a form of birth control. She has not used any form of birth control in the past and neither has her boyfriend. She also complains of a yellowish vaginal discharge, and has been wearing a panty liner to deal with this. Upon examination, Noelle complains of some abdominal tenderness, but denies that she has had any tenderness prior to this time. Noelle is screened for chlamydia and gonorrhea. She denies having had sex with any other partners, but does admit that she and her boyfriend had a fight and broke up temporarily about a month ago. They went back together about a week later. She does not know if he had any other sexual contacts during their period of separation.*

1. What other information should be elicited from Noelle?
    Ask Noelle whether she has had any dysuria, abnormal menstrual flow (and the time and character of her last menstrual flow), and whether she has noted any gray-white vaginal discharge.

2. What are the diagnostic tests that Noelle most likely received in the clinic to determine whether she is infected with chlamydia or gonorrhea?
    EIA or ELISA, direct immunofluorescence, culture of endocervical secretions

3. What other sexually transmitted diseases will Noelle most likely be tested for in addition to chlamydia and gonorrhea?
    She may be tested for syphilis, trichomoniasis, or HIV.

4. Write three nursing diagnoses and goals for Noelle.
    ***Nursing Diagnosis 1:* Knowledge deficit related to sexually transmitted disease.**
    ***Goal:* Noelle will state understanding of methods of transmission and treatment of gonorrhea and chlamydia.**
    ***Nursing Diagnosis 2:* Anxiety related to threatened sexual identity.**
    ***Goal:* Noelle will express feelings of anxiety related to her diagnosis.**
    ***Nursing Diagnosis 3:* Noncompliance related to shame and fear of diagnosis.**
    ***Goal:* Noelle will state understanding of treatment regimen and will return for her next visit as scheduled.**

5. List the medications that Noelle will be most likely to receive to treat a chlamydial infection.
    Medications include: doxycycline (Vibramycin) or azithromycin (Zithromax).

6. List some complications which Noelle may experience if she does not receive treatment for an active chlamydial or gonorrheal infection.
    There is a possibility of tissue inflammation, ulceration, scar tissue formation, infertility, salpingitis, and PID.

7. What information will you include when you counsel Noelle regarding sexual activity and forms of birth control? (See Chapter 31, Female Reproductive Disorders, for additional information.)
    Her partner must be treated concurrently. If she has unprotected sex with him, she may become reinfected. Barrier methods, the male or female condom, will need to be used until the infection is cleared up.

ANSWERS TO THE REVIEW QUESTIONS

1. When obtaining a health history from a client, the nurse asks the client to report on the presence of which of the following common symptoms of syphilis:
   d. painless sore or ulcer in the genital area
2. The two most effective medications commonly used to treat chlamydia are:
   a. doxycycline and azithromycin.
3. The organism responsible for the spread of the sexually transmitted disease, syphilis, is known as a:
   b. spirochete.
4. When instructing a client with gonorrhea regarding medication, the nurse will be sure to tell him:
   a. to take the medication until it is gone.
5. If a female client with chlamydia fails to complete treatment, complications that may arise in the future include:
   c. infertility and ectopic pregnancy.

CHAPTER 34

Digestive Disorders

SUGGESTED RESPONSES TO THE CASE STUDY

Ms. R. is a fifty-two-year-old female admitted to the hospital with acute abdominal pain. Ms. R. complains of right upper quadrant pain radiating to the back. She has had prior episodes, usually occurring about two hours after eating. This episode, however, is not resolving. Ms. R. also complains of nausea. Her vital signs are 152/88, pulse 92, and respirations 24 and shallow. Ms. R. is a slightly obese female who states she has recently been dieting to lose weight. Laboratory analysis includes a CBC with slightly elevated WBCs; bilirubin is elevated; and alkaline phosphatase is elevated. An IV is started and Ms. R. is given meperidine (Demerol) IM for pain. Ms. R. has been made NPO. An ultrasound of the gallbladder is ordered.

1. List subjective and objective data a nurse would want to obtain about Ms. R.
   Additional information should include dietary habits since the pain began, skin turgor, skin color, bowel sounds, response to pain to palpation, urine output, and urine color.

2. List risk factors other than those Ms. R. has that would put a client at risk for developing cholecystitis.
   Multiparous females, women on birth control pills, clients on Lopid, and clients with a history of small bowel disease such as Crohn's.

3. The gallbladder ultrasound show stones and an ERCP is ordered. What preparation will Ms. R. need for the procedure?
   NPO 6–8 hours prior to the procedure. PT, PTT, and bleeding time prior to the procedure.

4. List two nursing diagnoses and goals for Ms. R.
   Possible nursing diagnoses include:
   ***Nursing Diagnosis 1:* Pain, acute, related to inflammation.**
   ***Goal:* Ms. R. will verbalize increased comfort within one hour of analgesics.**
   ***Nursing Diagnosis 2:* Knowledge deficit, related to the ERCP.**
   ***Goal:* Ms. R. will verbalize understanding of the ERCP and postprocedure care.**
   ***Nursing Diagnosis 3:* Knowledge deficit, related to surgery.**
   ***Goal:* Ms. R. will verbalize understanding of the surgery and postsurgical care.**

Nursing Diagnosis 4: Fluid volume deficit, high risk for, related to NPO.
Goal: Ms. R. will demonstrate adequate hydration as evidenced by I&O nearly equal.

5.   The ERCP is successful in removing the CBD stone. The decision is made to perform a laparoscopic chole-cystectomy. What teaching will Ms. R. need?
Four small incisions will be made on Ms. R.'s abdomen. The gallbladder will be removed with a scope guiding its removal. She will be ambulated later in the day and will go home the next day. She will only be able to participate in moderate activity, such as walking, for two weeks.

6.   Why is meperidine (Demerol) the medication of choice for pain control?
Meperidine is believed to cause less spasms in the sphincter of oddi.

7.   List at least three successful outcomes for Ms. R.
(1) Discharge from the hospital.
(2) Adequate hydration level.
(3) No complications from procedures or surgery.

ANSWERS TO THE REVIEW QUESTIONS

1.   A client with a bleeding esophageal varix:
c. should have the Minnesota tube deflated every four hours.

2.   A client with a perforated duodenal ulcer:
b. may need to modify his or her diet after surgery.

3.   Clients with Hepatitis C:
a. should be instructed that all the mechanisms of transmission are not known.

4.   Changes in the digestive system caused by aging:
d. may require the client to swallow two to three times with each bite.

5.   Crohn's disease:
c. can be a debilitating disease leading to depression.

6.   Hernias are a protrusion through the muscle wall and:
c. can lead to bowel obstructions.

CHAPTER 35

Urinary System Disorders

SUGGESTED RESPONSES TO THE CASE STUDY

Ruth Andrews, fifty-six, is a client in the extended care facility. She has amyotrophic lateral sclerosis (ALS) with muscle weakness that has progressed and involves her legs and arms. A hydraulic lift is used to transfer her out of bed. A student nurse and a classmate enter with the lift to assist Ms. Andrews OOB, when she asks to use the bedpan. As they help her on the bedpan, they recall that the staff nurse gave Ms. Andrews the bedpan about a half hour ago. Returning in a few minutes, they help Ms. Andrews off the bedpan and notice the urine is cloudy with a foul odor. Ms. Andrews is not on I&O; however, they noticed that there is a very small amount of urine. She tells them that she does not know why she is going to the bathroom so often and why her urine smells bad.

1.   What subjective data should be gathered? What objective data should be gathered?
Any pain or burning when urinating? Does she feel she cannot wait when she feels the urge to urinate? Does she have a low-grade fever?

2. List diagnostic tests that may be ordered.
   A clean catch, midstream urinalysis with microscopic exam. Culture and sensitivity.

3. Write two nursing diagnoses for Ms. Andrews, related to her cystitis/UTI.
   Nursing Diagnosis 1: **Urinary elimination, altered, related to disease process as evidenced by having to urinate so often.**
   Nursing Diagnosis 2: **Knowledge deficit, related to signs and symptoms as evidenced by client comments.**

4. Write a goal related to each of Ms. Andrews's nursing diagnoses.
   Goal 1: **Ms. Andrews will return to usual timeframe of elimination.**
   Goal 2: **Ms. Andrews will verbalize understanding of signs and symptoms to report to the nurse or physician.**

5. List pertinent nursing actions for the care of Ms. Andrews for each of the following areas as they relate to the cystitis/UTI:
   Elimination, bladder: Have bedside commode for her use, she will be able to empty her bladder more completely than when using the bedpan.
   Diet and fluids: Encourage fluid intake of at least 2,000 mL/day with 1,000 mL being water and several glasses of cranberry juice each day.
   Safety, comfort, and rest: Check on Ms. Andrews at least every hour so that she knows you will be there. As the medications take effect, plan times for her to use the bedside commode so it will not be rushed and will be safer. She will be able to rest better then.
   Teaching: The importance of drinking the specified amount of fluids and cranberry juice. Report any dysuria or burning on urination.
   Nursing Staff: Check on Ms. Andrews every hour. Answer her call light promptly.

6. List two classifications of medications used for the treatment of an UTI.
   antimicrobials; urinary tract analgesics.

7. List two successful client outcomes for Ms. Andrews.
   (1) Ms. Andrews urinates every two to three hours.
   (2) Ms. Andrews tells you that if she ever has any burning or pain when urinating she will let you know.

ANSWERS TO THE REVIEW QUESTIONS

1. A client states she has had pain when urinating for three days. This would be documented as:
   b. dysuria.

2. A client has been admitted for chronic pyelonephritis. She is jittery and states she is concerned. Which of the following signs would indicate potential kidney damage?
   a. Urine output is 100 mL on your shift

3. Georgia Smithson has glomerulonephritis. This condition affects her:
   a. kidney.

4. Mr. Ronald Osborne, seventy-six, has had hematuria for several years and has been diagnosed with cancer of the kidney. His prognosis is poor. He told the nurse that he was too dizzy to go to the bathroom alone. Which of the following shows Mr. Osborne needs further teaching?
   c. refusal to wait for the nurse to lower the siderail.

5. Jake Jones, sixty-four, has had hematuria for several years. He is admitted to your same-day surgical unit scheduled for cystoscopic fulguration. Postoperatively, which of the following would you anticipate?
   a. blood in the urine

6. Lawrence Denny, twenty-nine, had impetigo two weeks prior to his noting a decrease in urine output and urine that "did not look right." His admission diagnosis is acute glomerulonephritis. He is on intake and output with fluid restriction. Which of the following comments indicates knowledge of his nursing care?
   c. "I put my call light on so you can empty my urinal."

7. Gael Dominich is a client with chronic glomerulonephritis. She is discharged home with home health care. As the LP/VN assigned to her case, you are planning Gael's A.M. care. While preparing the bath supplies, she says, "Please do not use any soap. My skin is so dry and flaky." The rationale for this would be:
   a. kidney failure leads to uremia.

8. Oliguria is best defined as:

    a. scant urine output.

9. Mr. Tom Surrey, in his fifties, is attending classes to be able to do his own peritoneal dialysis. He states he feels well and is eager to continue to learn. Mr. Surrey asks if washing his hands before the procedure is important. The best response is:

    b. "Yes, as you want to keep the procedure as clean as possible."

CHAPTER 36

Ostomies

SUGGESTED RESPONSES TO THE CASE STUDY

Mr. T.J. was admitted to the surgical unit after having an ileostomy with a total colectomy. His entire large intestine was removed due to ulcerative colitis. The incision is covered with a thick gauze surgical dressing, it is dry and intact. The stoma, on the right side of the abdomen, is pouched with an empty, two-piece transparent pouching system. The stoma is red and appears edematous.

Mr. T.J. has an IV of D51/2NS infusing at 125 cc per hour. There is a Jackson-Pratt drain from the lower right abdomen with a small amount of serous drainage in it, the bulb is compressed. He has a nasogastric tube connected to low, continuous suction. He is drowsy, and responds to his name easily. Mr. T.J.'s vitals are stable, he is comfortable, and his family seems supportive.

In the evening, after being medicated for pain, he stands by the side of the bed and marches in place. He is aware of his incision and notices that there is some yellow-green effluent in the pouch on his side. His first response is to make a face and look away.

In the morning Mr. T.J. asks his nurse if the stoma will always be so large. The nurse reassures Mr. T.J. that the stoma will shrink for the first six to eight weeks. As the nurse empties the yellow-green effluent from the ileostomy pouch, she explains the procedure in simple terms. Mr. T.J. looks away and does not seem to pay attention.

1. What assessment data in the case study would support the nursing diagnosis of altered body image?

    Mr. T.J. looks at his stoma makes a face and looks away. He asks if his stoma will always be so large. Mr. T.J. looks away and does not pay attention to the nurse's explanation of care. The client may not want to look at or think about the stoma, he may change the subject, or make jokes about not being normal anymore. The nurse needs to be sensitive to the client's wishes and acknowledge that this must be a difficult time for him. Help the client explore ways he may have used to cope in the past that might help in this case.

2. Which nursing diagnosis is most important for Mr. T.J. at this time?

    The most important issue for Mr. T.J. would be body image, altered. He needs to assimilate the stoma into his body image. The altering of the ability to control his stool elimination is difficult also and can be addressed under this nursing diagnosis. This can be a very difficult time for clients; they need much help and support from their friends and family. Some clients will have mood swings in an attempt to push others away, or answer the unasked question of how can you like me with this awful thing that has happened to me?

3. Develop a short-term goal for Mr. T.J. related to the nursing diagnosis in question 2.

    A short-term goal for Mr. T.J. would be: Mr. T.J. will look at his stoma, and begin self care of the ostomy, as demonstrated by emptying and changing the pouch with minimal assistance by discharge.

4. List three interventions that you could use in a care plan for Mr. T.J. related to the nursing diagnosis in question 2.

   (1) Allow Mr. T.J. to talk about what having this ostomy means to him and his lifestyle. Rationale: Will provide the client with an outlet to explore how his life may change and how it may stay the same.

   (2) Help Mr. T.J. identify support people he is close to who have made positive statements or behaviors after his surgery. Rationale: Will identify accepting behaviors of those close to Mr. T.J. as we draw our self acceptance from how others react to us.

   (3) Be positive in your approach to ostomy care with Mr. T.J. Smile when looking at the ostomy, do not look away, provide positive feedback about life with an ostomy. Rationale: People will look to the nurse and health care professionals to see how they react to the change in their body.

   (4) Arrange with Mr. T.J. for an ostomy visitor to come visit in the hospital. Rationale: Trained visitors can demonstrate that life after ostomy surgery is worth living and can be done.

   (5) Ask ET nurse to provide information for Mr. T.J. on living with an ostomy, and a visit to talk about what having an ostomy means to someone's lifestyle. Rationale: Identifies another support person and provides information on the benefits of having an ostomy over continuing the disease process of ulcerative colitis.

5. Develop outcome criteria for Mr. T.J. that could be used to evaluate your plan of care.

   Mr. T.J. is able to look at and change his ileostomy pouch with minimal assistance from the ET nurse. Mr. T.J. is able to get up to the bathroom and empty his own ileostomy pouch. Mr. T.J. states where he can find supplies and support when he goes home.

ANSWERS TO THE REVIEW QUESTIONS

1. On what would the nurse focus his assessment when a preoperative client is to have an ostomy?

   b. the client's knowledge and acceptance of surgery

2. Postoperatively, an ostomy client's pouch is starting to leak. What is the best action?

   b. Change the pouch as fast as possible since the client does not like to see the stoma.

3. Which of the following is an appropriate behavioral objective for a client with an urostomy prior to discharge?

   c. Change the appliance without assistance.

4. The ostomy client in room 300 is five hours postoperative. Assessment of his stoma reveals it is an edematous dusky to black stoma. What should the nurse do with this information?

   d. Cover the client back up and check the client in 30 minutes.

6. A client with a new ostomy asks his nurse on the first postoperative day, "Will this stoma be big and red like this forever?" What is the best response?

   c. "The stoma will always be pink to red, but that swelling will go down in six to eight weeks."

7. On the fourth day after surgery, a new ostomy client asks if he might be able to irrigate his ostomy. He has heard that some people do not have to wear pouches when they irrigate their ostomies. What is the best reply?

   b. "Irrigation to manage an ostomy is only done with colostomies or ostomies that have a storage segment of the bowel."

8. You are working when an ostomy client who was discharged two weeks ago calls from home to ask what she should do. Her husband went shopping and her pouch is starting to leak. What is the best suggestion?

   b. Use this opportunity to encourage her to change her pouch by herself.

Resources

CHAPTER 2:
LEGAL ASPECTS OF NURSING

Choice In Dying, Inc.
200 Varick Street
New York, NY 10014
212-366-5540

Medcom, Inc.
6060 Phyllis Drive
Cypress, CA 90630
800-877-1443

Living Wills
Films for the Humanities and Sciences
PO Box 2053
Princeton, NJ 08543-2053
800-257-5126

The Verdict Is:
Medical Electronic Educational Services, Inc.
930 Pitner Avenue
Evanston, IL 60202
800-323-9084

CHAPTER 4:
BIOMEDICAL ETHICS

American Red Cross
Transplant Services
800-2-TISSUE

Council of Regional Genetics Networks
Cornell University Medical Center Genetics, Box 53
1300 York Avenue
New York, NY 10021–4885

Nurse Genetic Specialists
International Society of Nurses in Genetics
3020 Javier Road
Fairfax, VA 22031

National Abortion Federation (consumer hotline)
800-772-9100 or 202-546-9060

National Society of Genetic Counselors
233 Canterbury Drive
Wallingford, PA 19086–6617

The Living Bank International
P.O. Box 6725
Houston, TX 77265
800-528-2971

United Network of Organ Sharing: UNOS
800-24DONOR

CHAPTER 5:
COMMUNICATION

American Health Information Management
    Association
919 N. Michigan Ave. Suite 1400
Chicago, IL 60611-1683
312-787-2672

CHAPTER 6:
CULTURAL ASPECTS OF
HEALTH AND ILLNESS

National Association for Spanish Speaking Elderly
2025 I Street NW, Suite 219
Washington, DC 20006
202-293-9329

National Asian-Pacific Center on Aging
Melbourne Tower
1511 Third Ave., Suite 914
Seattle, WA 98101

National Caucus of the Black Aged
1424 K Street NW, Suite 500
Washington, DC 20005

National Indian Health Board, Inc.
1602 S. Parker Rd., Suite 200
Denver, CO 80231

National Indian Council on Aging
P.O. Box 2088
Albuquerque, NM 87103

National Association of Hispanic Nurses
2300 W Commerce Suite 304
San Antonio, TX 78207
210-226-9743

National Black Nurses Association, Inc.
P.O. Box 1823
Washington, DC 20013
202-393-6870

CHAPTER 7:
CULTURAL DIVERSITY IN THE WORKPLACE

AT&T Language Line Services
800-752-6096 (over-the-phone interpretation of more than 140 languages)

National Association of Hispanic Nurses (NAHN)
202-387-2477

National Black Nurses Association (NBNA)
202-393-6870

Transcultural Nursing Society
313-591-8320

CHAPTER 8:
HEALTH MAINTENANCE

Aerobics and Fitness Association of America
15250 Ventura Blvd., Suite 310
Sherman Oaks, CA 91403
800-445-5950

American Dietetic Association
800-366-1655

American Health Care Association
1200 Fifteenth St. NW
Washington, DC 20005
202-833-2050

American Holistic Nurses' Association
205 St. Luis St. #506
Springfield, MO 65806-1317

Center for Science in the Public Interest
1501 16th Street, NW
Washington, DC 20036
202-332-9110

Centers for Disease Control and Prevention
Morbidity and Mortality Weekly Report
http://www.cdc.gov/cdc.html

Centers for Disease Control and Prevention
1600 Clifton Road, NE
Atlanta, GA 30333
404-639-3286

Clearinghouse for Occupational Safety and Health Information
Technical Information Branch
4676 Columbia Parkway
Cincinnati, OH 45226
800-356-4674
513-684-8326

Consumer Product Safety Commission
Washington, DC 20207
800-638-2772
800-638-8270 TDD
800-492-8104 TTD in MD only

Dental Disease Prevention
Centers for Disease Control and Prevention
1600 Clifton Road, NE
Atlanta, GA 30333
404-329-1830

Environmental Protection Agency
Public Information Center
401 M Street, SW
Washington, DC 20466
202-382-2080

Food and Drug Administration
Office of Consumer Affairs
5600 Fishers Lane
Rockville, MD 20857
301-443-3170
800-332-4010

Food and Nutrition Information Center
National Agricultural Library Building
Room 304
Beltsville, MD 20705
301-344-3170

Healthy America, National Coalition for Health Promotion and Disease Prevention
1015 15th St NW
Suite 424
Washington, DC 20005

Medic Alert Foundation International
P.O. Box 1009
Turlock, CA 95381
800-344-3226
209-668-3333

National Cholesterol Education Program Information
    Center
4733 Bethesda Avenue, Room 530
Bethesda, MD 20814
301-951-3260

National Council Against Health Fraud
3030 Baltimore St.
Kansas City, MO 64108
800-821-6671

National Health Information Clearinghouse
P.O. Box 1133
Washington, DC 20013-1133
800-336-4797

National Highway Traffic Safety Administration
Nes-11 HL
U.S. Department of Transportation
400 7th Street, SW
Washington, DC 20590
202-366-9294
Auto Hotline: 800-424-9393

National Institutes of Health
9000 Rockville Pike
Bethesda, MD 20814
301-496-4000

National League for Nursing
350 Hudson St
New York, NY 10014
212-645-9685
800-669-9656
Fax: 212-989-3710
e-mail: nlninform@nln.org

National Safety Council
444 N. Michigan Ave.
Chicago, IL 60611
800-621-7619

National Wellness Association/National Wellness
    Institute
University of Wisconsin-Stevens Point Foundation
South Hall
Stevens Point, WI 54481
715-346-2172

National Women's Health Network
514 Tenth Street, NW
Washington, DC 20004

Office on Smoking and Health
Technical Information Center
Park Building, Room 1-16
56 Fishers Lane
Rockville, MD 20857
301-443-1690

Poison Control Center
800-392-9111

President's Council on Physical Fitness and Sports
450 5th Street, NW, Suite 7103
Washington, DC 20001
202-272-3430
or
701 Pennsylvania Ave., NW Suite 250
Washington, DC 20004
202-272-3430

Sex Information and Education Council of the United
    States
80 Fifth Avenue, Suite 801
New York, NY 10011
212-673-3850

The Aerobics and Fitness Foundation
800-233-4886

The Institute for Reproductive Health
8721 Beverly Boulevard
Los Angeles, CA 90048
213-854-6375

The National Institute on Aging
P.O. Box 8057
Gaithersburg, MD 20898

U.S. Department of Agriculture
800-535-4555

U.S. Department of Health and Human Services
Office of Disease Prevention and Health Promotion
Washington, DC 20201
202-245-7611

World Health Organization
111 T.W. Alexamder Rd.
Durham, NC 27709
919-541-7537

CHAPTER 9:
SUBSTANCE ABUSE

Al-Anon
One Park Avenue
New York, NY 10016
800-344-2666

Al-Anon/Alateen Family Group Headquarters
P.O. Box 862
Midtown Station
New York, NY 10018-6106
212-302-7240

Alateen
One Park Avenue
New York, NY 10016

Alcoholics Anonymous (AA)
P.O. Box 459
Grand Central Station
New York, NY 10017

Alcoholism Center for Women
1147 S Alvarado Street
Los Angeles, CA 90006

American Council for Drug Education
204 Monroe St. Suite 110
Rockville, MD 20850
800-488-DRUG
301-294-0600

American Council on Marijuana and Other
  Psychoactive Drugs
6193 Executive Blvd.
Rockville, MD 20852

Cocaine Helpline
800-662-HELP

Codependents Anonymous (CODA)
P.O. Box 33577
Phoenix, AZ 85607-3577

Drug Abuse Resistance Education (DARE)
Local Police Department

Drug Enforcement Administration (DEA)
Office of Public Affairs
1405 I Street, N.W.
Washington, DC 20012

Families Anonymous
(Families of Substance Abusers)
P.O. Box 528
Van Nuys, CA 91408
818-989-7841

"Just Say No" Clubs
1777 N. California Blvd. Suite 200
Walnut Creek, CA 94596
800-258-2766

Mothers Against Drunk Driving (MADD)
669 Airport Freeway Suite 310
Hurst, TX 76053
817-268-MADD (6233)
or
311 Main Street, Suite C
Roseville, CA 95678
800-443-6233

National Association of Children of Alcoholics
31706 Pacific Coast Highway
South Laguna, CA 95677
714-499-3889

Narcotics Anonymous (NA)
World Service Office
P.O. Box 622
Sun Valley, CA 91352
818-780-3951

Narcotics Education and Rehabilitation Foundation
P.O. Box 4330
Washington, DC 20012

Narcotics Education, Inc.
Box 4390
6830 Laurel Street, N.W.
Washington, DC 20012

National Clearinghouse for Alcohol Information
Box 2345
Rockville, MD 20857
301-468-2600

National Clearinghouse for Drug Abuse Information
P.O. Box 416
Kensington, MD 20795
301-443-6500

National Clearinghouse for Smoking and Health
5600 Fishers Lane
Rockville, MD 20857

National Cocaine Hotline
800-COCAINE (262-2463)

National Council on Alcoholism, Inc.
12 West 21st Street
New York, NY 10010
212-206-6770

National Council on Drug Abuse
571 West Jackson Avenue
Chicago, IL 60606

National Drug Abuse Center
5530 Wisconsin Avenue, N. W.
Suite 1600
Washington, DC 20015

National Nurses Society on Addictions
5700 Old Orchard Rd. 1st floor
Skokie, IL 60077
847-966-5010

National Self-Help Clearinghouse
33 West 42nd Street
New York, NY 10036
212-840-1259

Office of Substance Abuse Prevention
5600 Fishers Lane
Rockwall II
Rockville, MD 20857
301-443-0373

Parent Resource Institute on Drug Education
100 Edgewood Avenue Suite 1002
Atlanta, GA 30303

Parents for Drug Free Youth
8730 Georgia Avenue, N.W.
Suite 200
Silver Spring, MD 20910
Hotline: 800-554-KIDS

Students Against Driving Drunk (SADD)
P.O. Box 800
Marlboro, MA 01752
617-481-3568

Toughlove
P.O. Box 10691
Doylestown, PA 18901
215-348-7090

CHAPTER 12:
PAIN MANAGEMENT

Agency for Health Care Policy and Research: Acute Pain Management Guidelines

Clinical Practice Guideline for managing acute pain. Available in three formats: (1) The clinical practice guideline (publication no. 92-0032); (2) Quick reference guides (Adults—no. 92-0019 and Pediatric—no. 92-0020); and (3) Pain Control after Surgery: A Patient's Guide (no. 92-0021)

AHCPR Clearinghouse
P.O. Box 8547
Silver Spring, MD 20907
800-358-9295

Agency for Health Care Policy and Research: Management of Cancer Pain

Clinical Practice Guideline for managing cancer pain. Available in three formats: (1) The clinical practice guideline (publication no. 94-0592); (2) Quick reference guides (Adults—no. 94-0593 and Pediatric—no. 92-0594); and (3) Patient's guide (no. 94-0595).

AHCPR Clearinghouse
P.O. Box 8547
Silver Spring, MD 20907
800-4-CANCER

American Pain Society

Principles of Analgesic Use in the Treatment of Acute and Chronic Cancer Pain, 3rd. ed. Skokie, IL: American Pain Society.

American Pain Society
5700 Old Orchard Road, First Floor
Skokie, IL 60077
847-966-5595

National Committee on Treatment of Intractable Pain
P.O. Box 9553
Friendship Station
Washington, DC 20016-1553
202-944-8140

Journals

The Journal of Pain and Symptom Management
Elsevier Publishing Co., Inc.
Journal Fulfillment Department
PO Box 882, Madison Square Station
New York, NY 10160-0200
Quarterly

The Clinical Journal of Pain
Raven Press Books, Ltd.
1140 Avenue of the Americas
New York, NY 10036
Quarterly

Pain
International Association for the Study of Pain
909 NE 43rd St., Suite 306
Seattle, WA 98105-6020
Monthly

Chronic Pain Letter
Box 1303
Old Chelsea Station
New York, NY 10011
Bimonthly

Organizations

American Pain Society
5700 Old Orchard Rd., First Floor
Skokie, IL 60077
847-966-5595

American Society of Pain Management Nurses
6437 S. Brooklyn Road, Suite A
Rochelle, IL 61068
815-378-0072

International Association for the Study of Pain (IASP)
909 NE 43rd Street, Suite 306
Seattle, WA 98105-6012
206-547-6409
Membership includes subscription to journal *Pain*.

National Chronic Pain Outreach Association
7979 Old Georgetown Rd., #100
Bethesda, MD 20814-2429
540-997-5004

National Committee on Treatment of Intractable Pain
P.O. Box 9553
Friendship Station
Washington, DC 20016-1553
202-944-8140

National Headache Foundation
525 North Western Avenue
Chicago, IL 60625
312-878-7715

National Hospice Organization
1901 North Moore St., Suite 901
Arlington, VA 22209
703-243-5900
Referral to local hospice: 800-331-1620

CHAPTER 13: PERIOPERATIVE NURSING

American Board of Post Anesthesia Nursing
 Certification
475 Riverside Dr.
New York, NY 10115
212-870-3169

American Society of Post Anesthesia Nurses
11512 Allecingie Parkway
Richmond, VA 23235
804-379-5516

Association of Operating Room Nurses
10170 E Mississippi Ave.
Denver, CO 80231-5711
303-755-6300

Second Surgical Opinion Program
200 Independence Ave. SW
Washington, DC 20201
800-638-6833

CHAPTER 14: FLUID, ELECTROLYTE, AND ACID-BASE BALANCES

National Kidney Foundation
30 East 33rd Street
Tampa, FL 33606
813-251-0725

CHAPTER 16: CARING FOR THE OLDER ADULT

Action
806 Connecticut Ave., NW
Washington, DC 20525
202-254-7310

Administration on Aging
330 Independence Avenue SW
Washington, DC 20201
202-245-0641

American Association of Homes for the Aging
1129 Twentieth St. NW Suite 400
Washington, DC 20036
202-296-5960

American Association of Retired Persons
601 E Street N.W.
Washington, DC 20049
202-434-2277

American Geriatrics Society
770 Lexington Avenue, Suite 400
New York, NY 10021
212-308-1414

American Society on Aging
833 Market Street, Suite 512
San Francisco, CA 94103
415-543-2617

Asociación Nacional por Personas Mayores
   (Hispanic Seniors)
3325 Wilshire Blvd., Suite 800
Los Angeles, CA 90010

Children of Aging Parents
1609 Woodbourne Rd. Ste. 302A
Levittown, PA 19057

Elderhostel International
75 Federal St.
Boston, MA 02110

Gerontological Society of America
1275 K Street NW Suite 350
Washington, DC 20005
202-842-1275

National Asian-Pacific Center on Aging
Melbourne Tower
1511 Third Ave., Ste. 914
Seattle, WA 98101

National Association of Area Agencies on Aging
600 Maryland Avenue SW, Suite 208
Washington, DC 20024
202-484-7520

National Geriatric Society
212 West Wisconsin Avenue
Milwaukee, WI 53203
414-272-4130

National Indian Council of Aging
PO Box 2088
Albuquerque, NM 87103

National Pacific/Asian Resource Association
2033 6th Ave., Suite 410
Seattle, WA 98121

CHAPTER 17: REHABILITATION, HOME HEALTH, AND LONG-TERM CARE

American Association of Homes for the Aging
Suite 400
1129 20th St. N.W.
Washington, DC 20036-3489
202-296-5960

American Association of Retired Persons
1909 K St. N.W.
Washington, DC 20049
202-872-4700

American Hospital Association
840 North Lake Shore Drive
Chicago, IL 60611
312-280-6000

American Health Care Association
1201 L Street N.W.
Washington, DC 20005
202-842-4444

Department of Health and Human Services
Public Health Service
National Institutes of Health
Bethesda, MD 20205
800-358-9295

Foundation for Hospice & Home Care
519 C St. NE
Washington, DC 20002

Health Care Financing Agency
200 Independence Ave. N.W.
Washington, DC 20201
202-245-6145

National Association for Home Care
519 C Street N.E.
Washington, DC 20002
202-547-7424

National Citizens Coalition for Nursing Home Reform
Suite L2
1424 16th St. N.W.
Washington, DC 20036
202-797-0657

National Rehabilitation Association
633 S. Washington St.
Alexandria, VA 22314

The Association of Rehabilitation Nurses
5700 Old Orchard Road, First Floor
Skokie, IL 60077-1057
847-966-3433

CHAPTER 18:
THE DYING
PROCESS/HOSPICE CARE

Association for Death Education & Counseling
638 Prospect Ave.
Hartford, CT 60105-4298

Concern for Dying
250 West 57th St.
New York, NY 10107

Foundation for Hospice and Home Care
519 C Street NE.
Washington, DC 20002
202-547-7424

Hospice Action
P.O. Box 32331
Washington, DC 20007

Make Today Count
101 1/2 South Union St.
Alexandria, VA 22314
703-548-9674

National Hospice Organization
Suite 901
1901 North Moore St.
Arlington, VA 22209
703-243-5900

CHAPTER 19:
RESPIRATORY DISORDERS

American Lung Association
1740 Broadway
New York, New York 10019
212-315-8700

American Thoracic Society
1740 Broadway
New York, New York 10019-4374
212-315-8808

Association for the Care of Asthma, Inc.
Spring Valley Rd.
Ossining, NY 10562

Centers for Disease Control and Prevention
Division of Tuberculosis Elimination
1600 Clifton Road
Mailstop E-10
Atlanta, Georgia 30333
404-639-2508

CHAPTER 20:
CARDIAC DISORDERS

American Heart Association
National Center
7272 Greenville Avenue
Dallas, TX 75231-4596
800-242-8721
http://www.amhrt.org

National Cholesterol Education Program
    Information Center
P.O. Box 30105
Bethesda, MD 20814-0105
301-251-1222
301-951-3260

National Heart, Lung, and Blood Institute
    Information Center
Public Health Service
P.O. Box 30105
Bethesda, MD 20824
301-251-1222

President's Council on Physical Fitness and Sports
701 Pennsylvania Ave. N.W.
Suite 250
Washington, DC 20004
202-272-3421

The Mended Hearts, Inc.
7272 Greenville Avenue
Dallas, TX 75231
214-706-1442

The Coronary Club, Inc.
9500 Euclid Avenue, E-37
Cleveland, OH 44195
216-444-3690

CHAPTER 22: BLOOD AND LYMPH DISORDERS

American Cancer Society (ACS)
1599 Clifton Road, N.E.
Atlanta, GA 30329
800-ACS-2345

Aplastic Anemia Foundation
P.O. Box 22689
Baltimore, MD 21203

Cancer Information Service (CIS)
800-4-CANCER

Center for Sickle Cell Disease
202-806-7930

Cooley's Anemia Foundation
105 E. 22nd St., Room 911
New York, NY 10010
800-221-3571

National Association for Sickle Cell Disease
4221 Wilshire Boulevard
Suite 360
Los Angeles, CA 90010
213-936-7205
800-421-8453

National Heart, Lung, and Blood Institute
9000 Rockville Pike
Bethesda, MD 20892
301-496-4236

Office of Cancer Communications
National Cancer Institute
Building 31, Room 10A24
Bethesda, MD 20892
800-4-CANCER

Sickle Cell Disease Foundation of Greater New York
1 West 125th Street, Room 206
New York, NY 10027

The Leukemia Society of America, Inc. (LSA)
733 Third Avenue
New York, NY 10017
800-955-4LSA
212-573-8484

The National Hemophilia Foundation
SOHO Building
Suite 406
110 Greene St.
New York, NY 10012
212-219-8180

CHAPTER 23: INTEGUMENTARY DISORDERS

American Burn Association
New York Hospital, Cornell Medical Center
525 E. 68th St., Room L706
New York, NY 10021
800-548-2876

American Hair Loss Council
100 Independence Place
Suite 207
Tyler, TX 75703
800-274-8717

Dermatology Foundation
1560 Sherman Avenue
Suite 302
Evanston, IL 60201-4802
847-328-2256

National Burn Victim Foundation
32-34 Scotland Road
Orange, NJ 07050
201-676-7700

National Institute for Burn Medicine
908 East Ann Street
Ann Arbor, MI 48104
313-769-9000

National Psoriasis Foundation
6600 SW 92nd
Suite 300
Portland, OR 97223
503-244-7404

Skin Cancer Foundation
245 Fifth Avenue
Suite 2402
New York, NY 10016
212-725-5176

CHAPTER 24:
ALLERGIES, IMMUNE, AND
AUTOIMMUNE DISORDERS

Arthritis Foundation
1314 Spring Street, NW
Atlanta, GA 30309
800-283-7800

Arthritis Information Clearinghouse
P.O. Box 34427
Bethesda, MD 20034
301-881-9411

Asthma-Allergy Hotline
800-624-0044
414-272-1004 in WI only (call collect)

Asthma and Allergy Foundation of America
19 West 44th Street
New York, NY 10036
202-265-0265
800-7ASTHMA

Lupus Foundation of America, Inc.
1717 Massachusetts Ave. NW
Suite 203
Washington, DC 20036
800-558-0121

Myasthenia Gravis Foundation
222 South Riverside Plaza
Suite 1540
Chicago, IL 60606
800-541-5454

The American Academy of Allergy and Immunology
611 E. Wells St.
Milwaukee, WI 53202

The American Lupus Society
260 Maple Court
Suite 123
Ventura, CA 93003
800-331-1802

CHAPTER 25:
HIV DISORDERS

AIDS Clinical Trials Information Service
1600 Research Boulevard, MS-1B
Rockville, MD 20850
800-874-2572

American Foundation for AIDS Research
733 Third Avenue, 12th Floor
New York, NY 10017
800-392-6327

American Red Cross
8111 Gatehouse Road
Falls Church, VA 22042
202-737-8300

Association of Nurses in AIDS Care
2500 NW 22nd St.
Miami, FL 33124

Centers for Disease Control and Prevention
Public Inquiries Office
1600 Clifton Road
NE Mail Stop A-23
Atlanta, GA 30333
404-639-3534

CDC: National AIDS Information Clearinghouse
P.O. Box 6003
Rockville, MD 20849-6003
800-458-5231

National Association of People with AIDS
1413 K Street NW 10th Floor
Washington, DC 20005
202-898-0414

National AIDS/HIV Hotline
c/o American Social Health Association
P.O. Box 13827
Research Triangle Park, NC 27709
800-458-2437

CHAPTER 26:
MUSCULOSKELETAL
DISORDERS

American Occupational Therapy Association, Inc.
P.O. Box 1725
1383 Piccard Drive
Rockville, MD 20849-1725

American Physical Therapy Association
1111 North Fairfax Street
Alexandria, VA 22314

National Amputation Foundation
1245 150th Street
Whitestone, NY 11357

National Easter Seal Foundation
70 E. Lake Street
Chicago, IL 60601

National Osteoporosis Foundation
1150 17th St. NW, Suite 500
Washington, DC 20036

Osteoporosis Foundation
612 N. Michigan Ave. Suite 510
Chicago, IL 60611

CHAPTER 27:
NERVOUS SYSTEM DISORDERS

Alzheimer's Association
919 N. Michigan Ave. Ste 1000
Chicago, IL 60611
800-272-3900

American Epilepsy Society
638 Prospect Avenue
Hartford, CT 06105-4298
203-232-4825

American Parkinson's Disease Association, Inc.
60 Bay St. Ste. 401
Staten Island, NY 10301
718-981-8001

American Spinal Injury Association
250 E. Superior Room 619
Chicago, IL 60611
312-908-3425

Epilepsy Foundation of America
4351 Garden City Dr.
Landover, MD 20785
301-459-3700

Guillain-Barre Foundation, International
P.O. Box 262
Wynnewood, PA 19096
215-667-0131

Huntington's Disease Foundation of America
140 West 22nd Street, 6th Floor
New York, NY 10011
800-532-7667

National Head Injury Foundation
1776 Massachusetts Avenue NW Ste. 100
Washington, DC 20036
202-296-6443

National Multiple Sclerosis Society
733 Third Ave.
New York, NY 10017
212-986-3240

National Parkinson's Foundation
1501 NW 9th Ave.
Miami, FL 33136
305-547-6666

National Spinal Cord Injury Association
600 W. Cummings Park Ste 2000
Woburn, MA 01801
617-935-2722

National Spinal Cord Injury Hotline
800-526-3456

Parkinson's Disease Foundation
William Black Medical Res. Bldg.
Columbia-Presbyterian Medical Center
650 W. 168th St.
New York, NY 10032
212-923-4700

CHAPTER 28:
SENSORY DISORDERS

American Academy of Ophthalmology
655 Beach Street
San Francisco, CA 94109
415-561-8500

American Council of the Blind
1010 Vermont Avenue NW, Suite 1100
Washington, DC 20005
202-467-5081
800-424-8666

Alexander Graham Bell Association for the Deaf
3714 Volta Place NW
Washington, DC 20007
202-337-5220

American Foundation for the Blind, Inc.
15 West 16th Street
New York, NY 10011
212-561-8500   620-2000

American Speech-Language-Hearing Association
10801 Rockville Pike
Rockville, MD 20852
800-638-8255

Association for Education of the Visually
   Handicapped
919 Walnut St. 4th Floor
Philadelphia, PA 19107

American Tinnitus Association
P.O. Box 5
Portland, OR 97207
503-248-9985

Better Hearing Institute
Box 1840
Washington, DC 20013
800-424-8576

Better Vision Institute, Inc.
1800 N. Kent Street, Suite 1220
Rosslyn, VA 22209
703-243-1528

Braille Institute
741 N. Vermont Avenue
Los Angeles, CA 90029
213-663-1111

Guide Dogs for the Blind
P.O. Box 1200
San Rafael, CA 94915
415-479-4000

Guide Dog Users, Inc.
12 Riverside St. Apt. 1-2
Watertown, MA 02172
617-926-9198

Guiding Eyes for the Blind
Yorktown Heights, NY 10598
914-245-4024

International Hearing Dog Inc.
5901 East 89th Avenue
Henderson, CO 80640
303-287-3277

Leader Dogs for the Blind
1039 Rochester Road
Rochester, MI 48063
810-651-9011

Lion's International
300 22nd St.
Oak Brook, IL 60521-8842
708-571-5466

National Association for the Deaf
814 Thayer Avenue
Silver Spring, MD 20910
301-587-1788 (TTY 301-587-1789)

National Association for Visually Handicapped
305 E. 24th Street
New York, NY 10010
212-889-3141

National Board for Certification
   and Hearing Instruments
National Hearing Aid Helpline
20361 Middlebelt
Livonia, MI 48152
810-478-5712
800-521-5247

National Society to Prevent Blindness
500 Remington Rd.
Schaumburg, IL 60173
312-843-2020
800-221-3004

Recording for the Blind, Inc.
20 Roszel Rd.
Princeton, NJ 08540
609-452-0606

Self Help for Hard of Hearing
4848 Battery Lane
Department E
Bethesda, MD 20814
301-657-2248

CHAPTER 29:
ENDOCRINE DISORDERS

National Institutes of Health
9000 Rockville Pike
Bethesda, MD 20892
301-496-4000

CHAPTER 30:
DIABETES MELLITUS

American Diabetes Association
ADA National Service Center
1660 Duke Street
Alexandria, Virginia 22314
800-232-3472
703-549-1500

American Association of Diabetes Educators
444 N. Michigan Avenue, Suite 1240
Chicago, Illinois 60611
800-832-6874
312-644-2233

Eli Lilly and Company
Educational Resource Program
P.O. Box 10B
Indianapolis, IN 46206

Juvenile Diabetes Foundation International
432 Park Avenue South
New York, New York 10016-8013
800-223-1138
212-889-7575

National Diabetes Information Clearinghouse
Box NDIC
9000 Rockville Pike
Bethesda, Maryland 20892
301-654-3327

CHAPTER 31:
FEMALE REPRODUCTIVE DISORDERS

American College of Obstetricians and Gynecologists
    (ACOG)
600 Maryland Ave. SW
Washington, DC 20024

American Fertility Society
1209 Montgomery Highway
Birmingham, AL 35216

Association of Women's Health, Obstetrical, and
    Neonatal Nursing (AWHONN)
1599 Clifton Road, NE
Atlanta, Georgia 30329
404-320-3333

Cancer Information Services
800-4-Cancer

Endometriosis Association
P.O. Box 92187
Milwaukee, WI 53202

National Breast Cancer Hotline
800-221-2141

National Osteoporosis Foundation
2100 M. Street N. W. Suite 602
Washington, DC 20037
202-223-2226

North American Menopause Society (NAMS)
Wolf H. Utain, M.D.
University Hospital of Cleveland
Dept. of OB/GYN
11100 Euclid Ave.
Cleveland, OH 44106

Older Women's League
730 11th Street, N.W.
Washington, DC 20001
202-783-6686

Women's Association for Research in Menopause
    (WARM)
128 East 56th St.
New York, NY 10022

CHAPTER 32:
MALE REPRODUCTIVE DISORDERS

American Association of Sex Educators, Counselors,
    and Therapists
11 Dupont Circle NW, Suite 220
Washington, DC 20036

American Cancer Society, Inc.
1599 Clifton Road, NE
Atlanta, GA 30329
800-ACS-2345

American Fertility Society
2131 Magnolia Ave., Suite 201
Birmingham, AL 35256
205-978-5000

Cancer Information Service
National Cancer Institute
Building 31 Room 10 A 07
Bethesda, MD 20892
800-498-3200

Impotence World Services
119 S. Ruth Street
Maryville, TN 37803

Recovery of Male Potency
Grace Hospital
18700 Meyers Rd.
Detroit, MI 48235
800-835-7667

RESOLVE, Inc.
5 Water Street
Arlington, MA 02174-4814
617-643-2424

CHAPTER 33:
SEXUALLY TRANSMITTED DISEASES

American Public Health Association
1015 Fifteenth Street NW
Washington, DC 20005

American Social Health Association
260 Sheridan Avenue
Palo Alto, CA 94306
VD National Hotline: 800-227-8922

American Venereal Disease Association
Box 22349
San Diego, CA 92122

Centers for Disease Control and Prevention
1600 Clifton Road NE
Atlanta, GA 30333
404-329-1388

National Foundation for Infectious Diseases
P.O. Box 42022
Washington, DC 20015

National Institute of Allergy and Infectious Diseases
National Institutes of Health
Bethesda, MD 20892

Planned Parenthood Federation of America, Inc.
810 Seventh Avenue
New York, NY 10019
212-541-7800

U.S. Department of Health and Human Services
Public Health Service
200 Independence Avenue, SW
Washington, DC 20201

World Health Organization (WHO)
Avenue Appia
CH 1211 Geneva 27
Switzerland

CHAPTER 34:
DIGESTIVE DISORDERS

American Anorexia/Bulimia Association Inc.
133 Cedar Lane
Teaneck, NJ 07666
201-836-1800

American Liver Foundation
1425 Pomptom Ave.
Cedar Grove, NJ 07009
800-223-0179

Bulimia/Anorexia Self Help
6125 Clayton Ave., Suite 215
St. Louis, MO 63139

Digestive Diseases Clearinghouse
1555 Wilson Blvd., Suite 600
Rosslyn, VA 22209-2461
(Includes PDQ search and information service)
800-4-CANCER

National Digestive Diseases Information
  Clearinghouse
P.O. Box NDDIC
Bethesda, MD 20892

National Foundation for Ileitis and Colitis
444 Park Ave. South
New York, NY 10016
212-685-3440

United Ostomy Association
36 Executive Park, Suite 120
Irvine, CA 92714

CHAPTER 35:
URINARY SYSTEM DISORDERS

Bard Urological Division
C.R. Bard, Inc.
Covington, GA
800-526-2687

Bladder Health Council
c/o American Foundation for Urologic Disease
300 West Pratt Street, Suite 401
Baltimore, MD 21201
800-242-2383
800-435-2732

Help for Incontinent People (HIP)
P.O. Box 544
Union, SC 29379
800-BLADDER

Medic Alert Foundation
P.O. Box 1009
Turlock, CA 95381-1009
209-668-3333

National Association of Patients on Hemodialysis and
    Transplantation
211 E. 43rd Street
New York, NY 10017
212-867-4486

National Kidney Foundation
30 East 33rd Street, Suite 1100
New York, NY 10016
212-889-2210

National Kidney and Urologic Diseases Information
    Clearinghouse
Box NKUDIC
Bethesda, MD 20892
301-468-6345

The Simon Foundation for Continence
P.O. Box 835
Wilmette, IL 60091
847-864-3913 (Headquarters)
800-23-SIMON (Patient Information)

United Network for Organ Sharing (UNOS)
3001 Hungary Spring Road
Richmond, VA 23228
804-289-5380

CHAPTER 37: GUIDELINES FOR INSTRUCTORS IN USING CRITICAL THINKING EXERCISES

The Foundation for Critical Thinking
4655 Sonoma Mountain Road
Santa Rosa, CA 95404

The Center for Critical Thinking and Moral Critique
Sonoma State University
4656 Sonoma Mountain Road
Santa Rosa, CA 95404
800-833-3645

Transparency
Masters

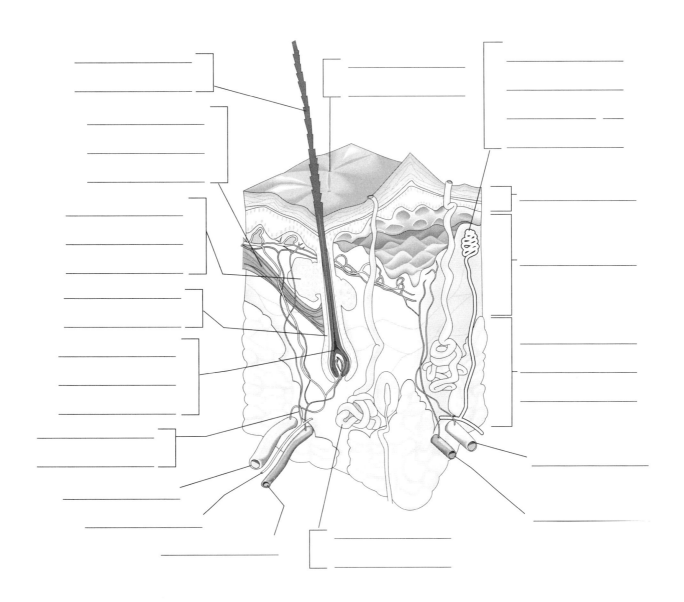

Posterior

Anterior

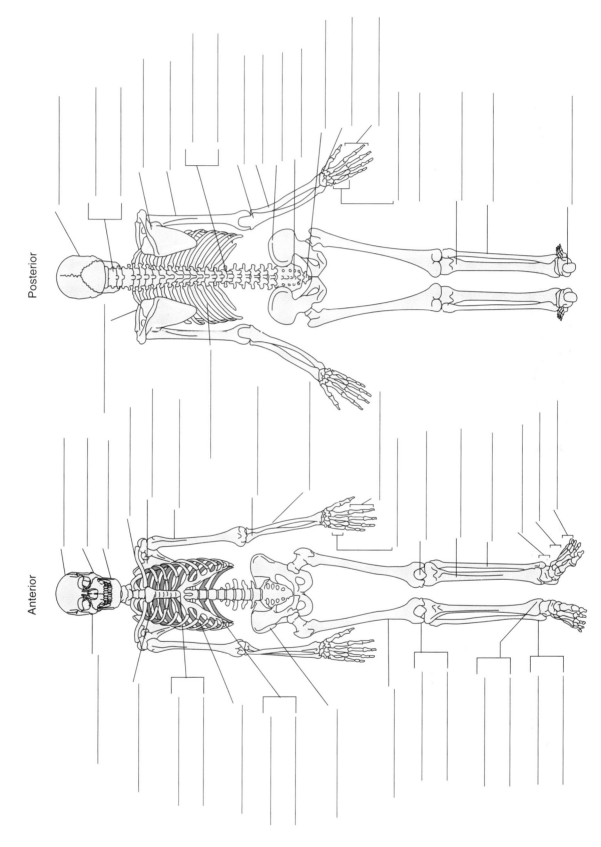

The Muscular System: Anterior and Posterior Views

Posterior

Anterior

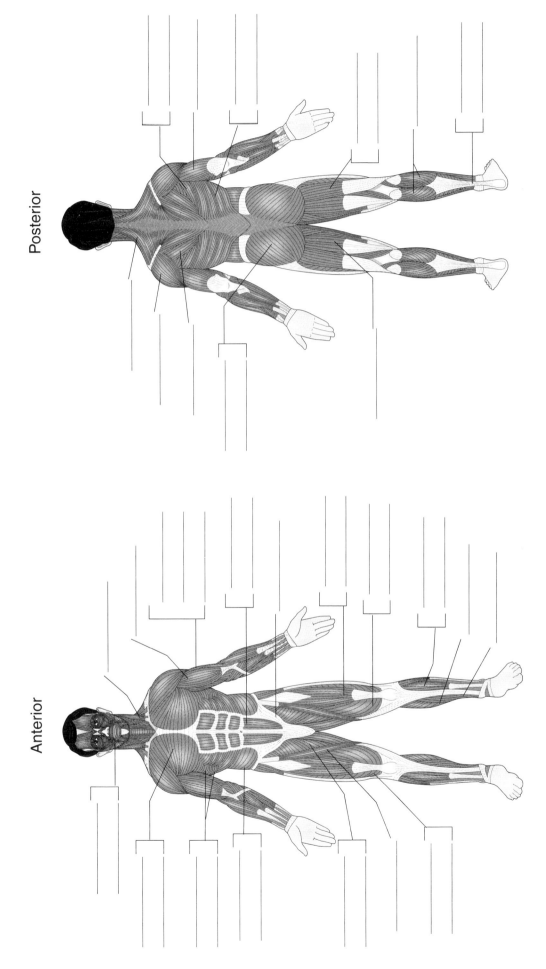

113

The Central Nervous System Includes the Brain, Spinal Cord, and Meninges

Structures of the Ear: Internal and External

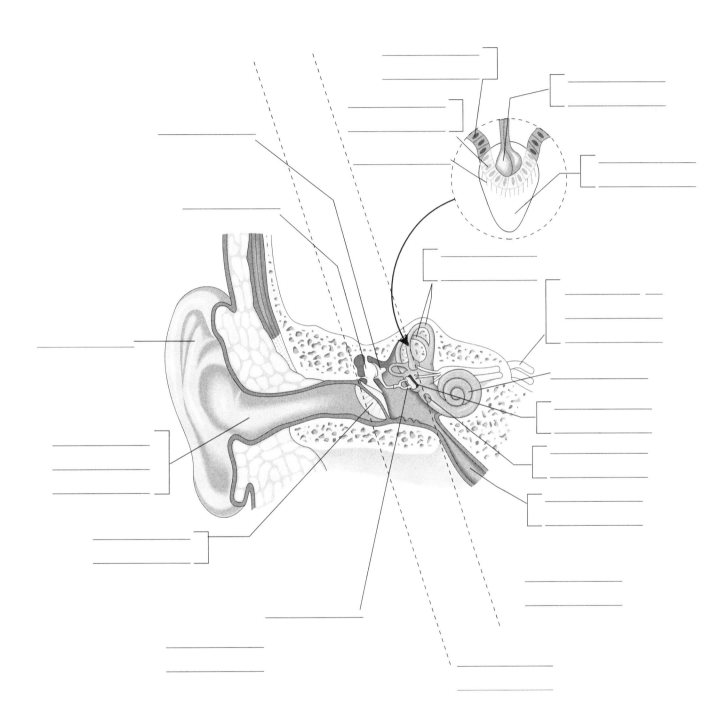

Lateral and External Views of the Eye

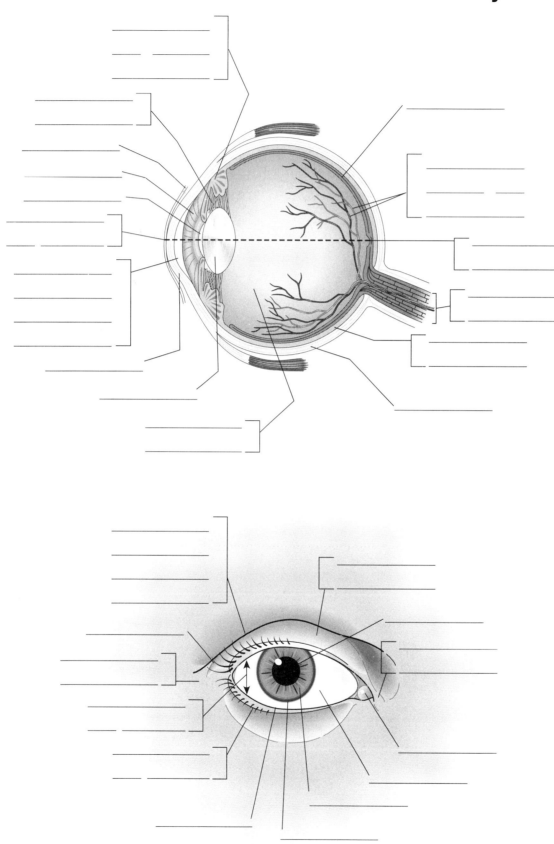

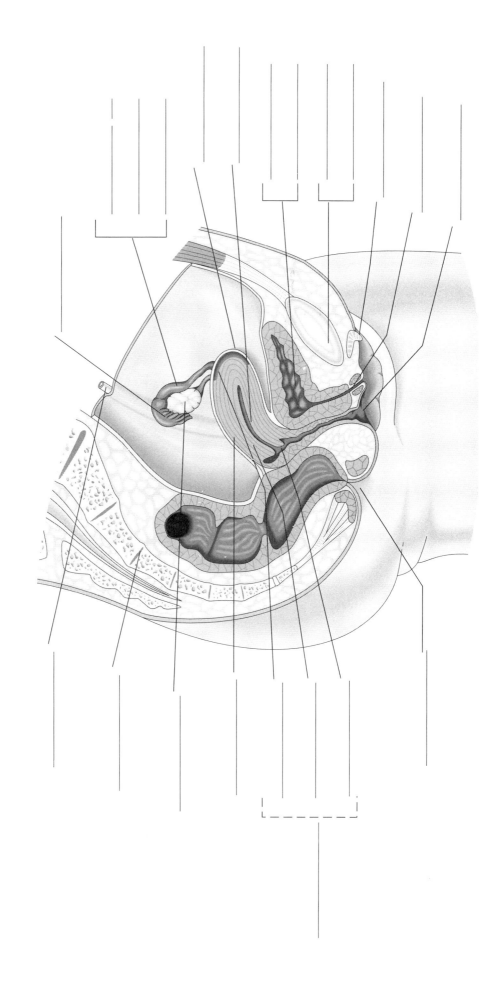

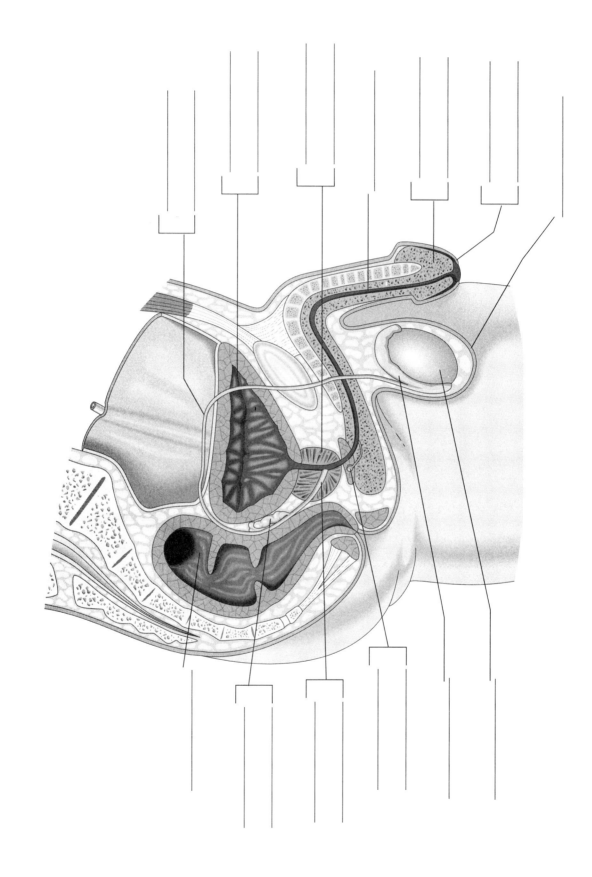

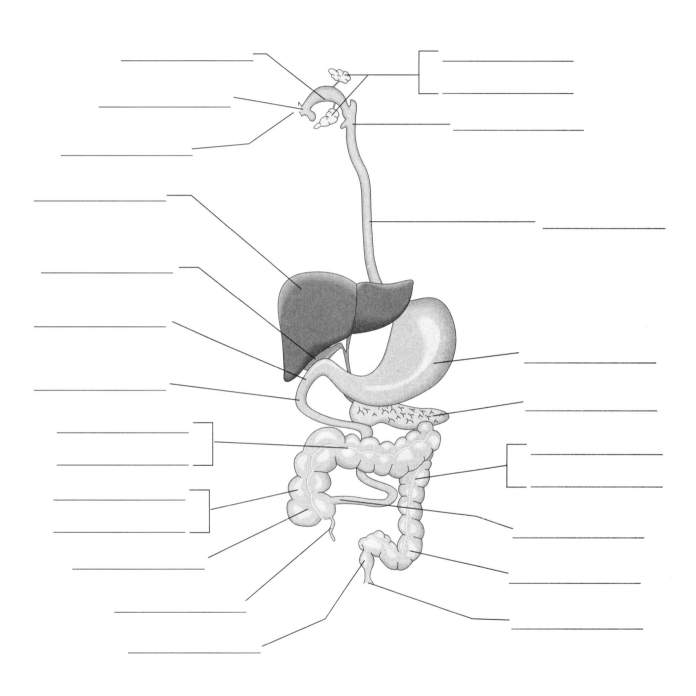

The Urinary System with Inset of a Nephron

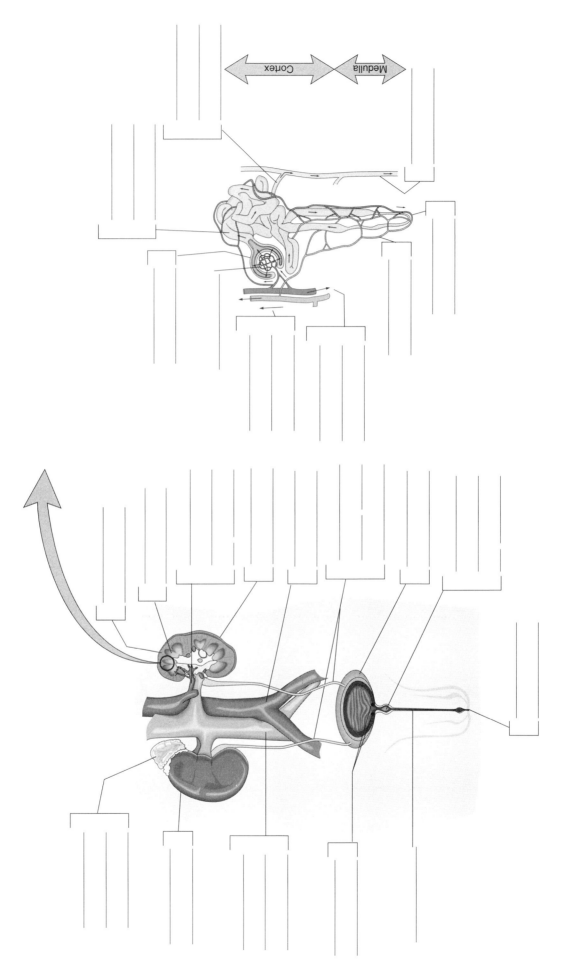

Cortex

Medulla